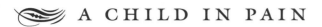 A CHILD IN PAIN

A Child in Pain

HOW TO HELP, WHAT TO DO

Leora Kuttner, Ph.D.

First Published by
HARTLEY & MARKS PUBLISHERS INC., 1996

Second Printing by
DR. L. KUTTNER, 2004

Library of Congress Cataloging-in-Publication Data
Kuttner, Leora
    A child in pain / Leora Kuttner.
      p.   cm.
    Includes index
    ISBN 0-88179-128-8
    1. Pain in children. 2. Child rearing.   I. Title.
  RJ365.92—dc20   96-13213
                       CIP

Designed and typeset by The Typeworks
Set in GALLIARD

Printed in CANADA

Dr. L. Kuttner
#204 - 1089 W. Broadway
Vancouver, BC V6H 1E5
Canada

CONTENTS

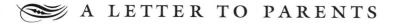 A LETTER TO PARENTS

DEAR PARENTS,

Having a child in pain can be one of the most distressing experiences of parenthood. I wrote this book to provide you with the latest information about pain and how to deal with a child in pain. This book is not intended to be a first aid manual, for there are many good ones already available, but rather a guide in responding to your child's pain and enabling your child to cope during painful episodes, to shift from being a victim of pain to gaining some mastery over the challenge of pain.

The many methods and medications discussed in this book will enable you and your child to cope with both minor and more serious pain from injuries or childhood and teenage diseases. The goal in working with pain, instead of fearing or fighting it, is to become "pain-literate," to be able to understand and interpret pain signals and to know what helpful actions ease pain. The guidelines in this book are meant to supplement the guidance and direction provided by your child's physician.

In this book, you will learn how

- to teach your child not to fear pain but to regard it as useful, something to be alert to;
- to help your child in pain;
- to understand enough about pain management and patients' rights that you can take steps to protect your child from unnecessary pain;
- to help your child use a range of coping strategies, rather than feel helpless when in pain;
- to learn about other techniques that provide pain relief to children;
- to learn about pain medication, its uses, benefits, and risks;
- to prevent pain in your child.

This book will also help you to talk with health care professionals in such a way that you will be listened to and not dismissed. As the first of its kind to address the social or interpersonal aspects of managing a child's pain, this book will give you the skills to create a truly cooperative relationship with health care practitioners to reduce your child's pain and distress and serve your child's best health interests.

Yours sincerely,

Leora Kuttner

A LETTER TO PROFESSIONALS WORKING WITH CHILDREN

DEAR COLLEAGUES,

When a child is in pain, all caregivers—including teachers, ambulance attendants, firefighters, daycare workers, police officers, nurses, doctors, child care counselors, physiotherapists, and blood technicians, among others—are in "loco parentis," and responsible for providing help and support to the child in pain.

Texts dealing with children in pain and trauma acknowledge that pain is multidimensional, that it is both an emotional and a sensory experience, but they do not offer enough information about children's pain and how to manage it. Steps are outlined for treating the wound or providing first aid, but the only guidance for coping with the effect of the pain on the child takes the form of "reassure the child."

Here is where this book starts. It provides you with language that will reassure the child, whether you know the child or not, and methods to help the child emotionally as well as physically. By clearly spelling out to the child what you, the child, or both of you together can do to manage the pain or help the pain settle, you can do a great deal to provide relief when a child is in pain.

Yours sincerely,

Leora Kuttner

INTRODUCTION

AS CHILDREN INVESTIGATE THE WORLD, they experience falls, bumps, and hurts of one kind or another, and they turn to their parents to find relief from pain. Pain is part of children's lives, yet we seldom if ever help parents to understand and manage such pain. Parents can play an essential role. Apart from providing comfort and relief, they can speak to a physician or other health care professional when a child can't express what is wrong. Parents are accurate judges of their child's pain and emotional distress. Parents are also the best source of information about what might be going on if the pain and distress are complex or continual. Most important, parents can raise children in ways that minimize the fear of pain, since fear worsens the experience of pain (Figure 1 shows the interaction of pain and anxiety which feed on each other in an upward spiral).

Some widely held historically based misconceptions about pain have prevented parents and professionals from dealing appropriately with children's pain. One of these is the myth of the split between mind and body. The concept that pain is either in the mind *or* the body goes back to the 17th-century philosophy of René Descartes, who argued that the body and mind were separate entities. He also maintained that there was a one-to-one correspondence between the injury and the amount of pain felt. Thinking this way about pain has retarded efforts to understand how our thoughts, feelings and behavior interact within our bodies to affect our perception and experience of pain. Splitting mind from body thereby limited our understanding of how to manage pain more comprehensively.

One of the earliest medical practitioners to publicly question this mind-body split was Dr. H. Beecher, a Boston surgeon who travelled to Europe with the U.S. troops during World War II. In 1956, he published a paper which described how soldiers who had very similar wounds to the civilians he had treated at home required less pain medications. In talking with these men, he realized that the meaning of their pain was very different from that for the civilian men. War wounds were a ticket home. Thus, the pain meant that the soldiers were out of active warfare. Beecher's reports challenged the simplistic thinking of the day and showed that the amount of tissue damage often bore little correspondence to the level of pain felt. These conclusions are now widely accepted. We now know that the meaning of a person's pain is subjective, highly personal, and variable from one situation to another, and that this meaning will influence how the pain is experienced.

Other research chipped away at the mind-body duality. In 1964, the Canadian psychologist Dr. Ronald Melzack developed the "gate-control" theory in his book *The Puzzle of Pain*. This theory proposed that the pain impulse from an injury could be blocked, weakened, or interrupted at points along the pain pathways to the brain by physical or psychological factors. Pain is not simply relayed along the pain routes, but can be regulated at many points ("gates") along the pain system pathways before *and after* reaching the brain. The "gate-control" theory radically changed our understanding of pain.

Until recently, health care professionals did not believe that children felt much pain. The medical reasoning was that infants and young children were immature neurologically, and therefore didn't feel pain in the same way as older children and adults. Children's screams in painful situations were believed to stem from fear, not pain. Yet, children as young as 15 months can let you know very clearly if it hurts or not. Newborn babies, as many parents know, are exquisitely sensitive to all forms of sensation, particularly pain. Any nurse on the nursery floor will confirm that even a premature 26-week infant will flinch and withdraw, or cry sharply when a heel of his foot is pricked to collect a small sample of blood.

Even when a child's pain could not be realistically denied, treatment was still withheld on the ill-founded grounds that the child would become addicted to opioids, such as morphine or codeine. Thus a child in pain after surgery did not get an adequate dosage of opioid. The undertreatment by professionals of children in pain was stunningly exposed in a pioneering study in Iowa in 1974, although at that time the finding had little impact. Dr. Jo Eland compared the medical charts of 25 children with those of 18 adults who had undergone similar surgeries. She found a startling and significant undertreatment of the children's pain, and a wide discrepancy in medication given to children compared to that given to adults. The common finding by other researchers in the 1980s was that medical and nursing staff, because of an ill-founded fear of addiction to opioids and the effects of opioids, gave young children and infants significantly less opioid medication than adults for similar pain conditions. In a landmark case in 1985 in Washington DC, Jeffrey Lawson was born prematurely and required heart surgery, common for premature infants. His parents were told that he would receive proper anaesthetic analgesia. Baby Lawson later died following cardiac surgery. Upon reviewing the chart his mother discovered he had received anesthesia and a paralyzing agent, but he had received nothing for pain. This case heightened public and professional awareness of the need to better understand infant pain assessment and management and that infants feel pain and require and deserve effective analgesia during surgery.

Twenty years after her first study, Dr Eland re-examined the pain treatment practices for children and adults in the same hospital. This time, children in pain received 968 doses of medication, compared with 24 in the earlier study. Clearly there has been an increased willingness to give children opioids, although attitudes and practices have not changed overnight—nor everywhere.

Recent medical research and the dissemination of information has begun to change professional views about the need to understand and manage infants' and children's pain. In 1986, the International Association for the Study of Pain formed the Special Interest Group on Pain in Childhood, to promote the study of children's pain and to educate the public and practitioners. Pain is now regarded as not merely a symptom of a disease, as had previously been thought, but as important as any disease. Clinicians and researchers are investigating how infants, children, and adolescents experience and respond to pain and what treatments are the most effective for the different ages. Physical, psychological and pharmacological methods of treating pain in newborns, young children, and adolescents are being developed. These methods have revolutionized the health care of children in hospital surgery wards and neonatal units and in the long-term treatment of painful medical conditions.

Now the fundamental principle of pediatric pain management is: *The child's pain is real and the child is the ultimate authority on this pain.* We are moving towards practices based on the belief that children are capable of being accurate witnesses, and need to be listened to and believed. Such thinking goes against years of practice in which health professionals have told children in pain "That doesn't really hurt", or "It can't be that bad!" or worse, "It shouldn't hurt." Whose body is in pain anyway?

Yet, in spite of our better understanding of the needs of children in pain, little effort has been made to take advantage of an interested and capable group of treatment allies—parents. It is extremely hard on parents to see their child in acute, persistent, or chronic pain and not to be able to do anything more than offer sympathy and reassurance. It is particularly hard for parents when their child has not been properly prepared for pain nor given adequate medication to provide pain relief. Parents can get caught between their natural urge to protect their child and the necessity for the painful medical treatment. Even worse for parents was the practice—seldom justified—of being required to wait outside the treatment room while the painful procedure took place.

This book is directed towards parents' natural desire to help their children. Because of what we now know about the intricate connection between the mind and the body, parents are in a position to take on the role of being the child's best ally in their times of pain. Parents, as their child's first teachers, can teach their child to become "pain-literate," just as they teach them to safely cross the road and manage other tricky situations. Clinical research and experience have shown that a basic knowledge of how pain is processed in the body, and how simple strategies of breathing, imagination, heat and ice, relaxation or hypnosis can help ease a child's pain and distress. Then children in pain can begin to develop mastery and skill, and gain some control of their own bodies, with their parents as their best coaches.

The idea of this book is not to make doctors out of parents. Neither is the book intended to take the place of a thorough medical investigation of a child's pain, nor should it replace a sound emergency or Red Cross manual. Rather the goal is to give parents and people working with children some skills and choices so that they can work cooperatively with each other in order to relieve pain and serve a child's best health interests. I also wanted to provide the sort of information and instruction that a multi-disciplinary team would provide to parents of a child in pain. To that end I invited colleagues from different disciplines to co-write chapters in their area of expertise. These are the chapters on medication (Dr. Christy Scott, a pharmacologist), emergency pain and the language that helps pain (Dr. Dan Kohen, a pediatrician), the use of TENS and acupressure (Dr. Jo Eland, a nurse), and dentistry (Dr. Penny Leggott, a dentist).

PART I

How Pain Affects Us
and Our Children

CHAPTER I

The Role Pain
Plays In Our Lives

PAIN IS PART OF LIFE. It plays an especially significant part in children's lives. Children frequently fall and scrape themselves as they learn to walk, run, climb, and ride a bicycle. They suffer accidents at home, in parks, in cars, and on the playground at school. They may experience pain when they get a tooth filled at the dentist's office or when they have an injection at the doctor's office. Some children struggle with painful diseases and hospital treatments. Parents and professionals working with children have a responsibility to teach children how to understand their painful experiences and how to manage their pain.

The Protective Value of Pain

In its healthiest form, short-term pain is protective, preventing damage and distress. As David, aged four and a half, discovered: "You've got to listen to your stomach when it's hurting, 'cause if you don't, your stomach will get upset!" David knew this firsthand; for five days he had had stomach pains and gastric spasms and had been throwing up. The pain signals had taught him that if he continued eating the tuna sandwich that his well-intentioned mother had given him, his stomach might send it back again.

David, who was recovering from a gastrointestinal virus, had come to respect the signals and sensations he was receiving from his stomach, which were helping him to eat only what his stomach could handle and telling him when to stop. Because his actions helped settle his pain and nausea, and because he was being listened to—although he was only four and a half—he was learning to manage his own distressing body experiences.

Children learn about their bodies when we encourage and teach them to pay attention to their bodies' messages and sensations, particularly pain. Children must learn how to interpret the different pain signals and to determine what gives the best form of relief. This learning becomes refined over an entire lifetime. Even very young children should be taught to become sensitive to pain signals, knowing what hurts, telling someone who is listening, and with that person determining what will help the pain to go and stay away.

We all want to avoid pain. In our society pain tends to be regarded with fear and terror. It makes us feel helpless, inadequate, vulnerable. Mostly, we would simply prefer not to deal with it. We want to shut it off, make it go away. Sometimes we minimize it. We become terrified when pain demands our attention, as if it has no right to be here at all, as if it isn't rightfully part of our bodies, our lives.

Yet pain offers vital information that guides us in the use of our bodies, tells us about the condition of our bodies, and helps us to survive. It is a rightful part of the workings of the human physiological system. We need to respect it and learn to work with it. It is our personal safety-alarm system, interpreted by our brains in a rapid, complex way. Pain messages quickly tell us about the status of our organs, muscles, bones, ligaments, and tissues, all of which are interwoven with nerve fibers that carry pain messages.

The value of pain can be seen when you consider people born with a congenital absence of pain, a rare condition in which one has an unusually high tolerance of pain. Throughout their lives, these people are at great risk of damaging their bodies. The absence of the protective feedback from pain signals to inform them of tissue damage puts these people in danger of major complications and injury. Pain does not protect them; it does not insist that they stop an action that will cause an injury or prompt them to call for help when they experience the early pain of an internal problem, like appendicitis.

Types of Pain

Pain comes in many different forms; David's pain, for example, was a dull warning pain. Pain is often generally categorized as acute, chronic, or recurrent.

ACUTE PAIN

Acute pain is pain associated with a brief episode of tissue injury or inflammation—for example, the pain caused by surgery, burns, a fracture, or a cut. Acute pain signals provide continuous, second-by-second sensory information. The pain begins suddenly, warning that tissue has been damaged, and usually lasts a short time. You know with extraordinary speed exactly where there is tissue damage or danger of further tissue damage. The pain sensation alerts you that something is wrong, mobilizing you physiologically and psychologically. Your brain receives the pain signal from the injury site as different chemical substances are released; your brain then releases substances, such as adrenaline and noradrenaline, that cause you to act to relieve the pain and return to some degree of equilibrium—for example, removing part of your body from danger or stopping what you are doing to minimize further harm. These actions occur reflexively and almost without thought. Pain shocks you into being protective. It is part of a marvelously sophisticated internal survival system that is highly effective, most of the time.

If children with acute pain—particularly when it is only mildly distressing—are encouraged to address their pain or distress promptly, relief will be more rapid. How the pain is described can lead to faster relief. Is that a sting or a tingling feeling, an ache or a sharp pain? Is it a big owie or a pinch? With guidance, children can learn to describe their pain more accurately, helping to clarify what is causing the pain and thus what treatment might be helpful. An ache such as muscle fatigue can respond well to heat or to a rub, rest, and analgesics. A burning or stinging pain may indicate inflammation as well as nerve injury and often feels better when an ice pack or a cool pack is applied and analgesic medication is taken. A sharp pain is a signal of more acute tissue damage, or it may indicate muscle spasm, such as the classic "stitch" in one's side while running. Relaxing the muscles by bending over from the waist and taking deep breaths will ease this pain. A dull, gnawing pain may indicate a more persistent pain, associated with ligament or tendon injury. Rehabilitation therapy or wearing a splint to restrain movement will ease this type of pain, giving the tissues time to heal.

Acute pain commands attention, causes anxiety, and drains energy. You remain uncomfortable and distressed unless this pain is adequately and effectively addressed. If the pain eases, you know your efforts have been successful. Generally, acute pain will diminish over a period of days or weeks, becoming less intense as time progresses. It is short-term and unlikely to return. Even though acute pain disappears, however, it can produce changes that linger in the body's nervous system. If not properly treated, these injured nerves continue to give signals and the pain will persist, becoming chronic or intermittently recurrent.

CHRONIC PAIN

Chronic pain tends not to be protective or informative but rather persists long beyond its initial useful or protective function. Examples of such pain are fibromyalgia, a rheumatological syndrome characterized by aching muscles and bones and specific tender points in the body; reflex sympathetic dystrophy, the experience of continuous nerve pain and hypersensitivity in a portion of a limb following trauma; and idiopathic pain, which means that the origins of the syndrome are not known, persisting beyond the initial injury or trauma.

Experiencing chronic pain is wearing and draining; it no longer serves to inform you of danger, which has long passed. Traditionally, chronic pain has been defined as pain that lasts longer than three to six months. But this definition does not describe the nature of the pain, which is often nearly constant, with few pain-free periods. Consequently, the pain becomes part of the person's life and hope is lost that it will ever go away. Without comprehensive treatment and therapy, people with chronic pain often feel that there is nothing they can do that will make this pain go and stay away.

Chronic pain often involves physiological changes to nerve fibers. Nerves that are damaged continue firing, or become hypersensitive to touch or pressure, even when the injury has healed. In chronic pain conditions and sometimes in conditions that have not had adequate pain relief, the involved nerves undergo physical and chemical changes. The nerves can become irritable and highly sensitive; often they do not respond in a predictable way to conventional medication or treatment.

Unfortunately, because chronic, persistent pain changes the way the pain system works, it often leads to more pain. These detrimental long-term neurological effects provide a compelling reason why children's pain must be promptly and adequately treated and controlled. Children with this type of pain may also have a physical disability from disease or trauma, which affects and limits all aspects of their lives. When a child suffers from chronic pain, the entire family must accommodate the child's increased needs, exacting an enormous toll in suffering and disruption for the child and family.

Children who have chronic pain can describe in impressive detail the quality, intensity, frequency, and subtle differences of the sensations.

Sixteen-year-old Jodi, who for five years struggled with a persisting nerve-muscle condition, experienced many different kinds of pain in the course of her very slow recovery. She became very sensitive to these different body sensations and learned to pay close attention to the distinctive characteristics of the pain signals she was receiving from her muscles and bones. They indicated important changes in her condition and, as a result, the treatment she would need. Over the years she became a fine and patient teacher of the doctors who would come onto the ward. When she was fifteen and was asked, "Do you have any pain?" Jodi explained that in fact she had three types of pain: "I have nerve pain, which is a shooting, sharp kind of sensation that comes sporadically and is not there all the time. Then I have muscle pain—I can't call it an ache, because an ache is something that you can put up with. It's more like someone has beaten you internally—it's a severe ache. My joint pain is like an arthritic pain, an osteoporosis kind of pain." Almost as an afterthought, she added, "The hard part was people not believing me!"

We need to let children know that we hear them when they are in pain and that we believe they are suffering. A body's pain system provides vital information about that body's well-being. We must learn to listen and to believe when anyone, especially a child, says he or she is in pain. For all of these reasons, children with chronic pain require a specialized long-term and intensive pain management program that involves changes in lifestyle, psychological treatment, physical therapy, and medication.

RECURRENT PAIN

Recurrent pain is pain that alternates with pain-free periods. Recurrent pains are far more common in children than are chronic pains, occurring in 5 to 10 percent of all schoolchildren. Common types of recurrent pain include tension and migraine headaches, abdominal pain, irritable bowel syndrome, and limb pains, which are fully discussed in chapter 8. Recurrent pains account for many missed days of school, and if a comprehensive treatment program is not quickly implemented, they can result in major disruptions in the school and social life of these otherwise healthy children. Like the treatment for chronic pain, the treatment for recurrent pain requires that the child actively participates in developing coping methods to assess and manage the pain over time. Treatment often needs to be a combination of pharmacological and psychological methods; each synergistically empowers the other, making the impact of the overall treatment greater.

Pain: The Mind and the Body

Not believing in another person's pain is in part due to the belief that pain is divided into physical and mental pain. David Morris, writer and physician, calls this the myth of two pains. According to the myth, there are two entirely separate types of pain: physical and mental. We are taught that these two forms of pain are as different as land and sea. Morris elaborates: "You feel physical pain if your arm breaks, and you feel mental pain if your heart breaks. Between these two different events we seem to imagine a gulf so wide and deep that it might as well be filled by a sea that is impossible to navigate." In fact, growing evidence indicates that there is continual interaction and intercommunication between our physical and mental functions, and that the division between physical and mental is an artificial construct that has retarded our understanding of the complexity of pain.

Pain is also an emotional experience. According to the official definition of pain provided by the International Association for the Study of Pain, "Pain is an unpleasant sensory and emotional experience associated with actual or potential tissue damage, or described in terms of such damage." Pain is experienced as emotional or mental suffering, as well as a distressing physical sensation, and it is subjectively experienced. It is private and entirely personal. In the words of sixteen-year-old Jodi, whose five-year experience of coping with severe pain from a neurological disorder qualifies her to instruct: "Pain is something that no one can analyze. How can you feel someone else's pain? You can't look at someone and say they are at an eight or a ten out of ten level of pain. How can you do that? It is internal; it's within that person. Only that person can say what level of pain they are in." She speaks the truth. We must ask individual children about the unpleasant sensory and emotional experiences associated with pain, guiding and helping them to assess, control, and relieve their pain. Working with pain is, however, not straightforward.

In every pain situation, however minor or severe, the interplay of our thoughts, beliefs, emotions, and attitudes with the sensations occurring in our bodies creates the experience of pain. This same interaction of mind and body enables us to increase or decrease pain sensations. However young a child is, with a plan and attention to the child's needs, pain can be eased and altered. Eight-year-old Seanna tells how this works for her during her regular but painful intravenous needles for cancer treatment: "I learned to use my imagination and go to a place I love—Candyland. I concentrate so much on what's happening there, that I don't even know there's a needle in my arm! It's funny how it happens. I just concentrate on Candyland and don't feel the needle!" Not all children can attain the level of concentration to turn off the pain entirely, but regular practice will maximize a child's natural coping abilities. Seanna reported that even when she was out of hospital, she practiced in the car while her parents were in the supermarket!

In contrast, 12-year-old Josh, a dramatic, highly imaginative young man, who detested coming into hospital, focused on all the awful things that could happen, and his fears were not constructively addressed. As a result, when Josh experienced a small pain, it quickly escalated into an overwhelming one. He concluded that if he imagined the worst scenario for himself, he would be prepared for any eventuality in hospital. So he imagined that he might die and worked himself up into such a heightened state of anxiety that his routine blood collection became a horrendous and painful experience for him, his family, and the staff. The instructions his mind gave his body were not "Shut down on the pain; it is an okay pain," but "ALARM! This could be my demise!"

Our mind and body also interact through the production and release of our own natural opioids, endorphins, not only in our brains, as first thought, but throughout our bodies. We now know that every major internal organ has its own opioid receptors. This means that every organ, including the gut lining, is designed to receive information in the form of chemical reactions from the brain, including the naturally occurring opioids for pain relief. Although we know that these internal pain relievers can be released through physical exercise, we do not know exactly how they are released—perhaps through relaxation, deep breathing, or meditation. It is possible that eight-year-old Seanna released enough endorphins to block the sensation of the needle in her arm, whereas Josh only succeeded in releasing large amounts of adrenaline to boost his panic and internal alarm.

Mixed Messages about Pain

Our society, in an attempt to deal with pain, gives many colliding and conflicting messages that often confuse the issues, while influencing our attitudes toward pain and our decisions about how to deal with pain.

PAIN AS A BATTLE

One message our society gives is to battle pain at all costs, to "fight the pain," as many advertisements advocate. Such injunctions promote an adversarial relationship with pain. The underlying but unhelpful ratio-nale goes something like this: *Pain is our enemy and must be beaten. In our fight against pain, tighten and tense up against these inner sensations.*

Because pain is seen as an enemy, fear prevails and panic reigns. Com-mon phrases like "This pain is killing me!" highlight the terror and life-threatening properties that we often give to pain. At times, pain reminds us of our vulnerability and even our mortality. In our battle to kill the pain within our own bodies, we pit mind against body. With this atti-tude we work neither intelligently nor compassionately with ourselves, and we do not use our mind-and-body network to promote relief.

The language commonly used to describe pain is the language of war. We rarely hear the notion of pain as friend, informer, or guide, aid-ing us to listen and use our bodies in gentler or wiser ways. We are taught instead that pain is an invader and an enemy. For relief against pain we are given "shots." Shots come from guns. They wound and hurt. No wonder children don't want anything to do with them! Some parents have used the threat of a needle to force obedient behavior from a child. Health care professionals have often heard a frustrated parent in a clinic saying to a wriggling, noncompliant child: "If you don't behave yourself, the doctor will give you a shot!" Most staff would promptly counter, "No, we're here to help you, not to punish you!" Nevertheless, the child has been instilled with fear and will remain distrustful—part of the legacy of war and threats.

In the battle against pain, television, magazines, and newspapers convey the message that you can arm yourself by relying on something outside of your body: a bottle of pills. The faces smiling with relief in advertisements are there to convince you that reaching for the pill is your only option. Rarely, if ever, are other options encouraged or taught, for it does not make much economic sense to teach a sufferer that actively using imagery or a relaxation tape, on its own or together with a pain medication, can control pain and discomfort.

PAIN AS BEING GOOD FOR YOU

Another message promoted in our society is that we must be stoic when we are in pain. According to this school of thought, pain is good for you, pain builds strength and character, and "pain will make a man out of you!" The motto "No pain, no gain" reflects this stiff-upper-lip attitude toward pain. The truth is that ignoring pain only adds to the strain of enduring it and depletes one's energy, joy, and vitality. When-ever pain is present, efforts need to be made to relieve it. Pain especially has no place in the lives of growing children; it is not needed for character, growth, or achievement.

The stoic ideal suggests that we should never use pain medication, or that we should feel shame or defeat when we do use it. "Endure the pain. Don't take anything for it. Don't give in!" we are admonished. Taking medication means weakness: you have lost the battle against pain. This position is also unhelpful in successfully managing pain. Medications given to a child in acute or persistent pain by a knowledgeable health professional will go promptly to the source of the pain and provide relief. Analgesics are, without question, the method to use when pain overwhelms and drains the child, as when a bone has been fractured, particularly when it is being set in a cast. Pain medication can also help in breaking a continuous cycle of pain, as when a child has a migraine headache. Medication provides the child with relief and a chance to sleep, to breathe more easily, and to use available energy to heal. When the child's energy has returned and the pain is no longer such a big issue, pain medication can be gradually withdrawn and other pain-reduction methods more heavily relied upon.

Controlling the pain promptly and keeping it well controlled is the fundamental principle of effective pain management to draw from these colliding and contradictory messages—that pain is a battleground in which fear reigns and medication is the only help, or that one must quietly endure pain to build character, since taking medication is a weakness. When pain is kept under control with adequate doses of pain medication, regularly given, less medication will be required than if smaller doses of medication are given at erratic intervals or only when the child's pain and suffering have become overwhelming.

Myths about Children and Pain

For many decades the myth that children don't experience pain has pervaded medical and nursing teaching and practice. A common response has been to ignore or underestimate a child's pain: "It's not really that bad. It can't be hurting *that* much!" Believing in these myths over many years has harmed children experiencing pain. The following case study reveals some of the long-term consequences of practices that neglect babies' and children's pain.

Rod, a 46-year-old police officer, is highly respected. He is decisive, physically tough, and capable on the job. Few people knew that vigorous Rod was born pre-

maturely. He spent the first four months of his life in an incubator and in a special care nursery, and had many painful medical procedures to aerate his lungs, feed him, draw blood, and check blood oxygen. Over the next five years, he had regular check-ups, which included blood tests and examinations. He has no clear memory of these early experiences, just his parents' stories. But Rod has one serious problem: he cannot stay in a room where there is a needle. Since the age of 12, he has never allowed blood to be taken without experiencing great trauma. He can't tolerate any invasive medical procedure. Try holding down a 230-pound man, let alone a man trained to fight! No blood technician, physician, or nurse had taken on the challenge.

Some unusual health difficulties forced Rod to consult a doctor, who said it was necessary to conduct a series of tests before making a diagnosis. Suddenly faced with either a serious health issue or a battery of medical tests, he needed help. Rod's terror was visceral and overwhelming: "I feel such a wimp. I can face and wrestle an armed man to the ground. But when a pint-sized nurse comes toward me with a needle, I clear out of the room! It's irrational. It's crazy!" No, it's not crazy at all. Rod had become sensitized at a very early age. He probably had not been given analgesics to control the pain before his many invasive medical treatments, since until recently it was believed that newborn babies did not feel pain. As a baby, he had experienced that there was nothing he or others could do to stop the pain. Now the mere idea of any medical procedure caused terror to overwhelm his 6'3" frame, and without knowing why, he would flee to safety.

Rod consulted a psychologist to conquer his deep, reflexive fear. He was ashamed of his fear and he wanted to learn how to desensitize himself to needles, how to manage that pain, and how to use his strengths in the other areas of his life to overcome this Achilles' heel. Highly motivated, he became skilled in using deep-breathing methods and self-hypnosis. After six weeks of graduated experiences with needles, in which he learned to regulate and lessen his own anxiety and to exercise his coping skills, he was able to have his blood drawn—a triumph!

If Rod's pain as a premature infant had been heeded and treated, he might not have developed an "irrational" terror. If, during the regular check-ups over his first five years, his fear had been noted and discussed with his parents and a plan giving him more control had been jointly devised, he would not have felt ashamed and powerless. There was much that his parents and the many health care professionals who treated Rod could have done to alleviate his pain. They could have supported him in learning how to work with the pain and not be frightened of it, thereby preventing his phobic reaction to medical interventions.

MYTH #I: NEWBORN INFANTS DON'T HAVE THE MATURE NERVOUS SYSTEM NEEDED TO EXPERIENCE PAIN

It has been maintained for many years that newborn babies are physiologically incapable of processing pain and that they are insensitive to pain. The rationale for this belief was that the physiological immaturity of infants—specifically, the lack of myelination (a protein sheath that surrounds the nerves and enables the nerve impulse to travel very rapidly) of the nervous system—meant that providing these babies with pain medication for painful invasive procedures was unnecessary. Newborns may not experience pain in the same way as an older child, since their nervous systems, including the brain, are still developing, but they are keenly aware of discomfort and react with distress to the pain from, for example, drawing a sample of blood from the heel. Over the last two decades, intensive research has demonstrated not only that newborns do experience pain but also that discounting their pain is far from good medical practice and is certainly not in their best interests.

We now know that from the middle period (26 weeks) of gestation, premature infants have developed central nervous systems to feel pain and the physiologic structures to transmit pain messages. Thus, the argument that the lack of myelination makes pain transmission difficult is totally invalid. Pain is transmitted over poorly myelinated and unmyelinated fibers, even in adults. Although pain messages are conducted more slowly in newborn babies, these messages have a shorter distance to travel.

Moreover, because the nervous systems of newborn infants are developing, they may not have the ability to modulate the transmission of pain signals and to exert control from the brain to the spinal cord. Thus, there is an increased chance that pain signals will persist in the babies' systems. The newborn baby may in fact feel greater discomfort than would an adult. Recent research in England suggests that newborn babies may have more available substance P (see p. 78) in the spinal cord than do adults, meaning that they have all the available chemicals to experience pain and, the research suggests, may even experience more pain than do adults. The newborn's exquisite sensitivity to pain combined with a lack of ability to modulate or shut down the pain signals, as can older children and adults, makes the pain management of newborns and babies imperative, especially for very sick babies in hospital care.

One example of the way we deny that newborns feel pain is the strong and pervading myth that circumcising a newborn infant is not painful for the baby. Many professionals, who are otherwise caring, compassionate human beings, are convinced that since circumcision has been practiced without anesthesia for centuries, and the baby cries for only 5 to 15 minutes, it can't really be painful.

In fact, evidence from controlled studies—such as the infant's immediate reaction to the surgery and increased irritability and wakefulness during the first hour following the circumcision—clearly indicates that circumcision performed without analgesia or anesthesia is experienced as painful by babies. Moreover, 90 percent of circumcised newborns show changes in behavior and greater difficulty in quieting themselves for up to 22 hours after the operation. These behavior changes are absent when babies are given local anesthesia for their circumcision.

Not very long ago analgesia and anesthesia for the newborn undergoing surgery were considered too risky. Witness these words from a surgery textbook written in 1938: "Often no anesthesia is required. A sucker of sugar water will often suffice to calm a baby." We now know that doing major or minor painful procedures without proper pain management is putting the newborn at even greater risk, increasing the baby's post-surgical complications and mortality risk and delaying healing and recovery, as well as being inhumane. Babies do metabolize opioids—the stronger analgesics recommended for surgery—much differently than do children and adults: babies' systems do not break the opioids down as quickly as children's systems. The analgesic thus remains in their blood longer, and the side effects can be greater and less predictable. Therefore, the pain management of infants and babies up to six or nine months of age requires nursing and medical expertise.

By approximately six months of age, babies show fear of painful situations, demonstrating a memory of painful events. Their nervous systems by this time have developed, so their response to pain is closer to that of the older child and adult than to the response of the newborn infant.

MYTH #2: CHILDREN DO NOT FEEL AS MUCH PAIN AS ADULTS DO

Children feel as much pain as adults do and perhaps even more. The underestimation of children's pain occurs especially in places where pain most frequently occurs, such as in blood collection laboratories. "Oh, this won't hurt," says the person giving, not getting, the needle. If the health care professionals do not respect a child's pain, understand the complexity of pain, or feel compassion for children, a child may hear the following remarks: "It doesn't hurt!" "Now, you don't have to be scared," "Oh, let's be brave," "Don't cry; be a big boy," and "It'll be over in a minute."

Isn't a minute of pain something to be rightly horrified about? A minute is an eternity for most children, particularly if the experience will be one of sharp pain. Sometimes there is at least a ten-minute period of waiting before the painful procedure will occur, but sadly there is no plan in place to address the child's fears ahead of time so that the pain won't feel as bad.

Insensitive remarks like those quoted above also reveal that the person does not appreciate the reality of the child's experience and does not realize that the child's fear of pain may directly affect his or her experience of the pain. Children all have their own ideas about the procedures done to them, and we only discover these ideas by asking. For example, six-year-old Stephan was upset about having blood drawn. When his mother asked him what was especially upsetting him, he answered by asking, "When they've taken my blood, will they give it back to me?"

Faced with having to perform painful procedures to help children recover and heal, professionals tend either to provide a supportive and understanding climate in which to do the procedure or to emotionally cut themselves off from the experience, acting merely as technicians and downplaying children's experience of pain. The latter individuals seem to have numbed themselves or built protective walls around themselves so that they don't need to address the emotional demands inherent in painful situations. Their attitude seems to be: "Let's just get it over as quickly as possible." Faced with this insensitivity, parents and other pediatric staff who can validate the child's feelings must speak up and be advocates for the child, creating a more manageable situation.

MYTH #3: CHILDREN WILL GET USED TO PAIN

Experiencing pain over time drains and debilitates children, as well as adults. Prolonged pain also causes changes in the nervous system, along with increased sensitivity and irritability. Thus, achieving relief becomes more and more difficult for children over time. Nor do children get used to acute or recurrent pain, such as the common and distressing experience of having an injection. The scientific evidence shows that children do not become used to needles with more frequent experiences of them. In fact, they often build up greater fears and learn to resist subsequent procedures unless a therapeutic plan to prevent this resistance has been developed for the child.

The anticipation of having another needle can disrupt a child's sleep, destroy the child's appetite, and make an otherwise normal child preoccupied, anxious, and clingy. Never underestimate the fear of pain. Once again, for adults as well as for children, *the fear of pain of a needle is often worse than the pain itself.* Children will go to great lengths to avoid pain. Sensitive nurses have been able to identify children who clearly are in pain because they're not playing or moving about in their usual way. When asked if they are in pain, some children have denied their pain because they suspect they'll be given a needle to make the pain go away!

A child who has had a bad experience with injections and has developed a fear of needles may show great ingenuity and desperation in bartering and negotiating to get out of receiving a needle. In extremes, a child has even hidden away on the ward or physically battled with medical staff to avoid the upcoming "shot." These extreme situations not only need to be avoided but must also be understood as the natural result of not providing the child with better ways of coping. At the very least, since the word "shot" carries an aggressive connotation, using the more apt term "injection" may remove the connotation of wounding.

MYTH #4: CHILDREN CANNOT RELIABLY EXPLAIN THEIR PAIN

Children are capable of reliably reporting their pain. If children are asked with non-leading questions where they hurt and how much they hurt, young children (even at 20 months) will answer by pointing to the site of their pain. With experience, even young children can become reliable interpreters of their pain signals. As six-year-old Jeffrey was chasing his older sister around the house, he slammed into the side of the dining room table. His father winced. "Oh, boy, that must have been a big hurt!" With a look that implied, "Well, really, Dad, you should know better," Jeffrey replied, "Dad, that wasn't a hurt; that was a whack!" "What's the difference?" asked his puzzled Dad. "Well, don't you know that a whack isn't serious? It's like a bump," said Jeffrey with authority. "But a hurt is serious, like when I cut my leg or when you bleed."

First, to explain their pain, children need to be asked where they are hurting. Second, the questions need to be in age-appropriate language, using words with which the child is familiar and comfortable. Third, the child must not feel overwhelmed or intimidated by the person asking the questions. If all three conditions are met, the child can become a helpful ally in the process of diagnosing the painful condition and monitoring progress with treatment. If the child feels she needs to please the person asking questions, however, the child may say what she senses the person wants to hear. When children feel intimidated by an authority figure, they are also likely to say something that does not convey a reliable picture. Younger children are more at risk for this than school-age children. Feeling intimidated or overwhelmed, however, indicates a problem in the clinician-child relationship and can be avoided if the child has a sense of comfort or a trusting relationship with the clinician.

MYTH #5: OPIOID ANALGESICS ARE DANGEROUS AND CAUSE ADDICTION

Fear of addiction is one of the reasons some people hesitate to use strong pain medications, such as opioids (the most common form of which is morphine). It is important to dispel this concern immediately, since it can hinder obtaining adequate pain relief. When a child is in severe pain, the use of opioids will not create an addiction. Unlike people who become addicts when they take drugs for recreation or pleasure, children (or adults) in pain do not become addicted when they take medication to combat pain.

Over time the child may indeed become more tolerant of the medication and greater levels may be required to relieve pain, but this is a physiological dependence, not drug addiction, which is a psychological as well as physiological dependency. Unlike substance abusers, children on opioids for pain relief are not psychologically dependent on their medication. They use the medication until their pain is no longer interfering with their lives. Treatment of a physiological dependence requires a gradual reduction in the medication to control withdrawal symptoms.

Using available pain reduction methods and medications with a child before or during a pain episode encourages the child's active participation in reducing the pain and fear and thus prevents feelings of victimization. Children will learn to become "boss of their own bodies" even when they are in pain. This goal, a central focus of this book, has not always been sought in child-rearing or pediatric practices.

MYTH #6: IF A CHILD CAN BE DISTRACTED, THE CHILD IS NOT IN PAIN

Distracting a child from pain—that is, shifting the child's attention away from the pain—in no way indicates that the child is no longer experiencing pain. It merely indicates that the child is capable at that moment of using his cognitive capacities to move away from the pain—a very useful coping method. It could also indicate that for that moment the pain did not absorb all the child's energy and was not all-consuming. Distraction does not exclude the existence of pain, however, and it cannot be used in that manner as a diagnostic tool. The golden rule is to ask the child if you are unsure whether or not the pain is persisting. The child's attention will then return to his physical sensation and the child will judge what is happening in his body.

MYTH #7: IF A CHILD SAYS HE OR SHE IS IN PAIN BUT DOES NOT APPEAR TO BE IN PAIN, THE CHILD DOES NOT NEED RELIEF

Pain is a subjective, private, and highly personal experience. Some children will openly exhibit their pain, some will hint at it, and others will cope by acting as if the pain were not there. It is therefore difficult to assess the presence or absence of another's pain merely by looking at the person. If a child says he or she is in pain, the child's pain needs to be attended to. The child is asking for help, and we must respond promptly and with compassion. The child does not need to convince us through certain behaviors of the existence of the pain; the child is the authority on whether or not he or she is in pain. Our job is to help.

Table 1.1 represents a summary of the common myths about childhood pain, now refuted by scientific evidence.

Table 1.1 Common Myths and the Scientific Evidence

Myth	Scientific Evidence
1. Newborns don't have the mature nervous system needed to experience pain.	By 26 weeks, a fetus in utero is capable of experiencing pain. At birth a newborn is highly sensitive to pain.
	Even though a newborn's nerve fibers are not fully myelinated, pain messages are still transmitted, and the newborn infant is well able to feel pain.
2. Children do not feel as much pain as adults do.	Children feel as much pain as adults do and perhaps even more.
3. Children will get used to pain.	Continuing pain has deleterious effects and causes long-term changes in the nervous system.

Myth	Scientific Evidence
4. Children cannot reliably explain their pain.	If asked, and listened to, children are capable at a very young age (even at 20 months) to say where it hurts, how much it hurts, and what helps the hurt feel better.
5. Opioid analgesics are dangerous for children.	Opioid analgesics are powerful pain-relieving medications that are invaluable for children in pain.
6. If a child can be distracted, the child is not in pain.	Momentary distraction does not exclude the existence of pain.
7. If a child says that he or she is in pain but does not appear to be in pain, the child does not need relief.	The child is the authority on whether or not he or she is in pain. If the child says, "I am in pain," the pain needs attention.

The Role of Crying

Crying is one of the ways we know when children are in pain, but as they grow society's attitudes toward crying often confuse and complicate this natural emotional and physical release. Crying is a way of releasing inner tension and distress in one's body. Children often spontaneously respond to their pain by crying, and they in turn are responded to in different ways, depending on their age, their sex, and the social implications of the situation. Whether we are aware of it or not, we all carry certain beliefs and attitudes about the display of emotion, particularly crying, and convey these attitudes to our children from early on in life. Some of the beliefs we learned as children are: "Crying is okay in private only," "Crying means you're weak," "It's okay to cry at weddings or funerals," "To cry is humiliating," "Big boys don't cry" (implying that you're really little if you cry), "Girls can cry, but boys have to be brave," and "If a boy cries, he's a sissy." All cultures and societies have well-defined attitudes about whether crying is allowed and under what circumstances and what crying means at those times. In most cultures, girls are given greater freedom of emotional expression than boys.

Crying is a natural and automatic response to pain. Tears release the physiological tension produced by trauma and pain. From birth, babies are able to cry spontaneously in connection with all forms of distress, such as feeling hungry, feeling unsettled, or being in pain. When a baby feels distress, her body tenses, her lips or jaw trembles, her eyes squeeze tightly together, her mouth opens wide, her tongue becomes taut and cupped, and she emits sobs of different degrees of intensity, which, together with deep inhalation and howling exhalations, release the tension from pain and discomfort and alert the baby's caretaker. Even the fact that crying can be exhausting can contribute to the relief of distress, for often after crying a baby will fall asleep. Hunger cries are higher pitched than pain cries and become more like pain cries if the infant is not fed — being hungry can indeed be painful. Over time parents learn to identify the sound of their infant's pain cry and facial expression of pain. Crying therefore has survival value as a distress signal, for it is the most immediate way that parents and caretakers are alerted that their baby is in pain.

Crying is increasingly inhibited or repressed as most children grow up. But adults do harm when they disapprove of children's tears. If a child is told that it is not acceptable to cry, his or her ability to express distress in a natural and healing way is impaired. Because of the powerful ways in which cultural beliefs and child-rearing practices entwine, the issue of how crying should be handled is a controversial one. There are, however, a number of things we know about crying.

1. *In general, children do not like to cry.* They don't feel good about crying, and if there is a choice in a situation, most psychologically healthy children prefer not to cry, whether it is physiologically relieving or not. School-age children and adolescents, in particular, are very concerned about "losing it"; crying represents failure and potential humiliation. Conversely, learning how to manage these difficult situations and to control the distress and pain becomes a worthwhile challenge and growing step for many children. If they successfully manage the pain and they don't cry, they experience an increase in their self-esteem and feelings of competence.

2. *Children in pain need the opportunity to express their feelings clearly.* We need to acknowledge our children's emotions, not only those of pain but also those of anger, fear, joy, envy, meanness, appreciation, or sorrow. When adults say disapprovingly, "There is nothing to cry about!" or "That doesn't hurt; now stop your crying," they are not promoting the child's developing sense of self or encouraging more effective coping; rather, they are denying the child's feelings. It is central to a child's emotional health that his experience be acknowledged and affirmed. Through an adult's acceptance and affirmation of the child's emotions, the child can learn for himself to know and develop his own identity. The young child's emotions and internal sensations form the

nucleus of the developing self. This nucleus is the beginning core and the point of crystallization of an emerging sense of self.

3. *In contrast, telling a child that "it's okay to cry" when the child is about to face a painful situation carries a message that may be unhelpful.* Many years ago, when it was not as acceptable to cry in public as it is today, physicians in training were taught that a sympathetic response to imminent pain would be to tell the child beforehand that it was okay to cry. Telling a child that it is okay to cry might indeed be helpful and supportive if the child has already spontaneously dissolved into tears and is feeling embarrassed, or if parents are trying to quiet the child because they think he or she is creating a scene. The physician's response of "It's okay if you need to cry" would be sympathetic and supportive of the crying child and instructive to the parents that a child's spontaneous crying is acceptable.

Telling a child who is about to have a painful procedure that it is okay to cry, however, conveys a very different meaning. It could mean, "What I'm about to do will make you cry, so if you do, it's okay!" What a statement of doom. Most children will immediately feel awful and may begin crying because there clearly is no way out. Parents and health care professionals must pay close attention to the messages encoded in the language they use.

In conclusion, pain plays a vital role in informing us about what is going on in our bodies and in keeping us healthy. Unfortunately, we live in a society that regards pain with fear and terror and holds the misconception that there are two types of pain: physical and mental. We now know beyond doubt that both mind and body are essential to experience pain, and that through the intricate interaction of mind and body, pain is increased or relieved.

CHAPTER 2

The Crucial Role of Parents

The Shift to Family-Centered Health Care

HISTORICALLY, HEALTH CARE WORKERS have not allowed parents a central role in the care of their child in pain. Nevertheless, parents, quite rightly, have insisted that they help manage their child's pain. Major changes are occurring in ideas about how health care should be provided, how much it should cost, and how it should be managed. A shift from a service model to a family-centered model has already occurred in pediatric hospitals. A cornerstone of this change is a new regard for parents, who are now seen as:

- the experts on their child
- a resource in caring for and managing their child's health; and
- partners in decision making and future planning.

These principles apply directly to managing children's pain. Parents are an invaluable aid in assessing, observing, and understanding the child's behavior. As mediators between the child and other adults, who don't know the child as well yet have to provide the child with medical attention, parents play a pivotal role in ensuring that this experience is beneficial for the child. Parents encourage the child to follow through with medical programs and interventions, such as taking medications, having blood collected, practicing self-hypnosis, and using biofeedback or music to ease chronic pain and illness.

Often parents must provide care that used to be provided by hospital staff. Children are being discharged from hospitals earlier and earlier after illness or major surgery to be cared for by their parents at home, with or without home nursing support. Surgical procedures such as the removal of tonsils and adenoids that used to require a child to remain in hospital for a few days following surgery are now routinely done as day surgery. Parents are having to assume more and more of the responsibility, care, and management of their children in pain as health care dollars continue to shrink.

Only 20 years ago, parents would take their child to a health care professional and the child would be taken away for treatment. Those days are gone. Gone also are the days when parents handed over their child for medical treatment and were not permitted to remain in the room. (The notable remaining exceptions are emergency and life-threatening interventions.) The 21st-century philosophy of "parents as partners-in-care" will also encourage health care professionals to re-assess their current practices for dealing with pain and to develop even more effective coping skills to help children in pain. In the next few decades parents will be regularly included and consulted as members of the diagnostic and pain-treatment team. With such a crucial role, parents will need to learn more about the dynamics of pain and about how to enable their children to develop flexible, non-fearful ways of coping with pain.

PARENTS AS ROLE MODELS

Children experience and observe how their parents deal with pain, talk about pain, and cope with pain. They continually learn from their parents' comments and responses to their own pain, their spouse's pain, and other children's pain. For example, after a tough day working at the hospital, I returned home complaining about how sore my head was. A few hours later my son, then aged three, came into the room holding his head, using the same words I had and complaining about his sore head. I was stunned. I realized I needed to be more thoughtful about demonstrating how to take care of my sore head and to put into practice what I teach. I invited my wriggly son to lie down on the bed with me, and together we put our heads on the soft pillows so that the pain could drain away. The lesson: All children, particularly young children, are masters at the powerful process of observational learning. They will absorb their parents' values, attitudes, and behavior toward pain, with or without our being aware of it. Not only will children demonstrate behavior toward pain similar to that of their parents but they will also convey the same fears and attitudes about treatments. A parent's belief about the effectiveness of a pain treatment can have a major influence on how the child will respond to the treatment. The parent's belief will determine the child's expectations for success and may influence how effective the results will be. For example, when parents tell their child that any treatment for pain other than medication is "hocus pocus," they impede the success of that intervention. In contrast, if parents tell their child how they used breathing methods and imagery during the child's birth, and how much that helped to get through the pain of the contractions, then the child knows that Mom and Dad will support his efforts to make it work for him too.

Four-year-old Pamela, a strong-minded and determined little girl, had acute lymphatic leukemia, which required regular intravenous chemotherapy into her hand. This occurred before the topical local anesthetic EMLA *(see pg. 178) was released for use with needles, and she understandably detested the procedure. With each treatment, she fought and resisted more. To enable her to have an easier time, Pamela and her mother were taught to make the skin on Pamela's hand go numb before she had her intravenous needle, using the hypnotic procedure known as the "magic glove" (demonstrated in the educational videotape* No Fears, No Tears; *for details see* Recommended Resources). *Her mother followed the directions and caressed her daughter's hand, covering it with the magic glove. She talked calmly and confidently to her little girl, saying that her veins had become much stronger, that they could now easily stand up, and that she wouldn't feel much or be bothered, because the magic glove was protecting her. Feisty Pamela delighted everyone by responding quickly and wholeheartedly. She concentrated on blowing and on the good, safe feeling of the magic glove. She watched intently, as if it were someone else's hand, as the needle easily went into her vein. With considerable insight her mother commented: "I had to show her that this can work, and I got right down to it with her. If I had said, 'Oh, this is junk!' or shown her that I didn't believe or agree with it, it would not have worked."*

Parents and staff have considerable impact on children's behavior before, during, and after stressful medical procedures. When, during painful medical procedures, adults help their children cope by using distraction, humor, and conversation not related to the procedure, the children themselves respond with coping skills, such as deep breathing. Even children assessed as having low coping skills respond by coping when an adult prompts them with commands such as "Breathe!" rather than with reassurance, apologies, and empathy. When adults respond with distress, such as apologizing, both high-coping children and low-coping children become distressed. Adults should be taught to promote coping, and children can and should be taught how to cope and to remain responsive to adults' coping prompts. It is encouraging to know that we can help a child cope by conveying that the painful situation is manageable and that telling a story, talking, or doing deep breathing will help the child get through it.

In contrast, the attitude that pain is punishment or a source of "justice" will not promote coping, because these beliefs tend to isolate and victimize the sufferer. (Giving pain a moral force complicates both assessing and treating pain and is hard on everyone.) The pain-as-punishment-or-justice motif is often expressed in words such as "It's not fair that . . ." "What did I do to deserve this?" or "I don't deserve this at all! After all I've done—to be punished in this way." When parents with the attitude that pain is some form of punishment experience their own pain, they tend to become grouchy and angry and to show resentment. They may become depressed because they feel bad, judged, or helpless. Such parents may make such statements as the following to their children: "It serves you right for . . ." "If you don't behave yourself, I'll give you something to really cry about," or "If you don't sit still, you'll get another shot!"

Removing this unnecessary moral judgment on pain can free both child and parent to deal more effectively with pain: "You didn't get this pain because you were bad. You are a good kid. It was [choose one] an accident/infection/inevitable because your family has this gene. Many people learn how to manage and get on top of this pain, and we'll support you to do that too, even if it feels very tough right now." These attitudes and coping patterns are learned early in life—the most powerful learning place is your own parents' home!

Our Inherited Belief System

Parents sometimes report being shocked at how in a crisis of pain they find themselves automatically repeating their parents' words. They never intended to say those words, perhaps because they had not found the words helpful when they were younger and in pain. Yet, in the height of a crisis, out they pour (which can be rather unsettling!). It is helpful to become conscious of these early behavior patterns and attitudes and to judge whether they fit you, your child, and your current situation.

Since your own early experience of pain and the manner in which you were raised to deal with pain affects your response to a child in pain, take a few moments to recollect what those early pain experiences were and what influence they have had on your attitude toward your child's pain. Below are some questions that could increase your sensitivity to your own reactions to pain, your partner's, and both your families' responses to pain. An increased awareness of these patterns can free you to make better choices about how to deal with pain.

From your parents' experiences with pain:
- How did your parents respond when they were in pain?
- How did each of your parents respond when the other was in pain?
- What did your parents do or say to you when you were in pain?
- How did you feel about their response?
- What are your family stories about being sick or being in pain?
- What were acceptable and unacceptable expressions of pain?
- Could you summarize your family's message about pain?

From your own experiences with pain:
- How do you deal with pain?
- Is your style similar to or different from your partner's?
- What do you consider your best ways of coping with pain?
- Why are they best for you?
- How has that affected the way you deal with your child in pain?
- What is your family's message about pain?

From your children's experiences with pain:
- How does your child deal with pain?
- What does your child do that you consider coping?
- How do you generally respond to your child's coping responses?
- Are you satisfied with how these responses work for you and your child?

Knowing more about the attitudes and dynamics of your family can help you make better decisions when a pain situation arises.

Which Parent?

If both parents are available when a child is in pain, which one would do a better job of supporting or coaching the child through a painful episode or procedure? In most parenting relationships, jobs are distributed in such a way that each adult deals with what she or he does best. This distribution evolves over time. Children in the family intuitively know about this distribution of labor. A child will know, for example, that Mom is the real disciplinarian or that Dad hates the sight of blood, even though he is great as the decision-maker about plans when some-one is sick. Commonly one partner functions better in certain crises than the other. Thus, a child will approach one parent rather than an-other about certain problems. The same applies to helping your child cope with pain. If both parents have experience and feel competent, ask the child whom she would like with her when she deals with her pain.

One family, whose eight-year-old daughter, Leanne, required frequent blood work and IVs, found that Leanne's mom was the better of the two parents to ac-company her into the clinic. Leanne's dad, a lawyer, related well to the staff, but when his daughter became distressed, he would turn into a tiger, fume at the nurse, and, in the confusion of his feelings, end up yelling at his daughter, who was already in tears. His response to her pain was deep rage that as effective as he was in the world, he couldn't stop his daughter from hurting. In contrast, al-though Leanne's mom had a sensitive stomach and easily became queasy, she was able to talk quietly and encouragingly to her daughter through her whimpering while the nurse found a vein. When she felt waves of nausea coming over her, she would fix her eyes on her daughter, take deep breaths to ease the queasiness, and say to herself, "If this little kid can go through this, I can too!" After practicing this way over successive treatments, Leanne's mom said that her concentration and focus on her daughter had strengthened, becoming quite intense. "It was like I was sending my power to her. The building could have fallen down and I wouldn't have known!"

Sometimes children do not have the luxury of choosing the more helpful parent for the situation. Parents work and have other children and daily demands. In these situations children should choose a favorite relative, adult friend, or grandparent. Being with the person who gives the child the most strength or supports him in the way he feels best can be very beneficial. Not only can it help to make the painful experience more toler-able and manageable, it can also deepen a significant relationship, which then becomes an extra resource for the child outside of his nuclear family. Grandparents have been powerful in this role for some children undergo-ing pain. Their greater life experience and wisdom are easily conveyed to the child by loving caresses or familiar stories. Grandparents thus create a calming, deeply comforting atmosphere for their grandchild.

Parents' Role as Teachers

Not only are these pain patterns passed from one generation to another but learning to make sense of the inevitable pains, both trivial and serious, starts early in a child's life. Parents tend to be the key people to explain and interpret confusing and alarming pain signals. Whatever their individual temperament, babies, toddlers, preschoolers, and school-age children continually and spontaneously learn from their key caretakers, absorbing information almost like sponges. The early years particularly are a high-intensity learning opportunity for establishing healthy attitudes toward pain.

When children are young, many parents and grandparents spontaneously offer to kiss a child's acute and sudden pain, to help the pain go away. Adults have used this warm and often effective response with distressed children, from infants to pre-adolescents, across many cultures. When alerted by a child's cries that he has hurt himself, a caring adult immediately runs over to the child to provide relief from the pain. This prompt response does in fact help the child in distress. The scenario with a child under ten years of age in a situation of acute but mild pain often runs something like this:

Child: (sudden burst of howls or crying)
Parent: (startled) What's happened?
Child: (crying) I hurt myself.
Parent: (quickly going over to the child) Oh dear! Do you have an owie? Let me see (examines injury and makes a pronouncement, for which the child has been waiting). This injury doesn't look too serious. Let's put a Band-aid on — the hurt should go away soon. Here, let me kiss it better. (The diagnosis will determine the child's subsequent reaction.)

The child continues to cry, but with lessened intensity. He is glad for the attention and comfort and for the reassurance that the sharp pain does not indicate something terrible, even though it feels terrible. Parents sense this and often give the child another hug, or hold the child before obtaining the Band-aid. After the comforting kiss, contact with parents, and the applied Band-aid, the child with tear-streaked face is able to dismiss his pain and readily returns to his play again.

Trust, reliance, and understanding, an implicit contract between child and parent, develop with many such experiences, over months and years . The parent's accessibility, quick response, and offer to "let me kiss it better" convey the clear message that "with a kiss, the hurt will begin to get better." Just as in fairy stories where a kiss has magic properties — as when a kiss wakes the princess — in real life a kiss takes the pain away. Having experienced this wonder before with a parent, the child feels comforted and trusts that it will work again.

Why the Child's Pain Diminishes

It is not only the child's belief but the flexibility of the child's entire pain system that allows the sudden and mild pain to diminish. At the onset of pain, the brain receives the signals and sends an "all-system alert" message. The parent's soothing words change the meaning of the pain from terrible to okay, thus altering how the pain is processed in the brain. The message travels through the brain, spinal cord, and peripheral nervous system that this pain signal, though sharp and distressing, is not life-threatening and will go away. Knowing that this is an "okay pain that will be better" allows rapid changes throughout the nervous system that inhibit and lessen the intensity of the pain signal. The brain is pivotal to all pain perception and behavior.

As in the example above, without necessarily knowing exactly what is happening in the child's brain, we notice from the child's expression and behavior that the child seems in less pain and is no longer alarmed. In time, the child may confirm our observations that he is no longer hurting. Here is one of the puzzles of pain: pain can only be inferred from a person's words or behavior. We can never experience other people's pain, nor can we measure it objectively, like temperature or heart rate. We can feel with them, and for them, but we can never feel or see their pain directly. Pain is a subjective experience. Thus, we need to ask, "Are you in pain?" The child's answer becomes the starting point; observations by others add to the child's statement of the quality, intensity, nature, and spread of the pain to provide a more comprehensive understanding of the pain experience.

The better we know another person, the better we are at gauging the level of pain. Knowing a child's temperament and behavior patterns and the meaning of his cry helps adults more accurately assess the kind of pain the child is experiencing. Observation, however sensitive and acute, can never replace the need to ask the child direct questions about his or her experience, such as:

- Are you feeling any pain?
- What kind of pain is it?
- How bad is the pain?
- What would help the pain to go?

The child's answers, together with our observations of changes in the child's mood, movement, and behavior, lead to an assessment of the child's pain and a decision about methods and medications to make it better.

Early Pain Training

Over months and years, if actively guided, children can learn to make sense of their body signals, not merely to respond to the hunger signals to eat, or the bowel and bladder signals to defecate or urinate, but also to call for help when there are pain signals and some part of the child's body doesn't feel right. Children can gain enormous confidence from their parents in making sense of and dealing with their distressing pain. Here a young child in pain demonstrates his assessment skills by giving the emergency physician his own diagnosis:

Four-year-old Clarence was brought to the emergency department of a children's hospital with a dislocated elbow. His naturally assertive mother briskly walked in and told the attending nurse the circumstances that led to his elbow being sharply pulled and dislocated. Clarence was in pain and unable to bend his arm. Somewhat tense, he held onto his mother with the other arm. The physician on duty examined his arm carefully and then pronounced, "This looks like a pulled elbow!" "No it's not!" said an amazed Clarence. "It's a swollen hand!" His forthright remark encouraged the physician to take the extra minute of valuable time to explain to Clarence in greater detail about the mechanics of his arm and why it caused him pain. This was important information for a curious child—in fact for any child. Clarence appeared to have modeled his mother's assertiveness in coping with his painful elbow, however tense he felt in the emergency department.

Developing confidence and authority about one's body is an essential part of developing into a well-rounded and competent person. Even at 18 months toddlers show clearly that they are aware of and sensitive to pain in their own and others' bodies. Toddlers are easily alarmed and sensitive to any threat to the integrity of their bodies. This was brought to my attention when I was on the floor with 18-month-old Narjit.

Narjit noticed a dime-sized hole in my stocking. With distress and consternation she pointed her chubby little finger at the hole and chimed, "Owie-owie!" She was alarmed by the hole. She seemed to be asking if it was hurting me, a possibility that clearly worried her. It was important to explain and to show her in a playful way that this owie didn't hurt me, that it belonged to my stocking and was painless. She then took some delight in repetitively poking her finger in and out of the hole, in the way toddlers play when they are attempting to master and come to terms with something. She was obviously relieved that this injury was not part of my body and did not hurt me—an early sign of her developing empathy.

With continual parental coaching, children can change their previously fearful responses to pain. Over time, depending on the nature and degree of exposure to painful experiences, children do develop ways of modulating, coping with, and changing these pain signals to regain an inner equilibrium and a feeling of well-being. Such development may seem to happen overnight when it coincides with other developmental milestones.

Jason, a rapidly growing five-year-old, who only months before wailed and demanded immediate attention whenever he hurt himself, stunned his mother as he landed flat on his face in the playground, skinning his hands. "Don't worry, Mom, it's only a scrape!" he called out from the gravel. What was the difference this time? wondered his mother in amazement, as she stopped herself from her usual run to his rescue. Was it the other children present? But they were always around. Was it his stronger sense of self-confidence now that he had just turned five and had begun kindergarten? Or was the change in his behavior due to the chats they had had about the muscles, the skeleton, and the messages the body gives? She was not sure if it was one or all, but she was thrilled that Jason was beginning to manage his occasional pain in a way that made both him and her feel good. He's growing up, she mused.

Helping Define the Meaning of the Pain

During a child's experiences of pain, parents also help the child to make sense of the pain, to give it a name, and to "put it in its place" so that it doesn't become a source of fear and worry. For example, after 16-month-old Chloe caught her chubby finger in a drawer, her mother said to her: "Your finger is sore? How did you hurt it? Did you catch it in the drawer? No wonder it's hurting! It is sore—but it won't last. Let's rub it to help the hurt to go. Here's a big hug. You can let the sad feelings go. It's okay now. Your finger is getting better already. I guess it isn't a good idea to play with the drawers. Instead, play with these boxes. You can put lots of things inside and your hands can't get caught. It's safe, so your fingers may like these boxes a lot more."

Children also need consistent coaching to learn how to deal with their pain, particularly if the pain persists or recurs, such as a headache. However young a child is, learning to understand and work with these internal sensations is an empowering process.

Four-year-old Tyler had migraine headaches. He would become irritable, whine, and be clingy. Initially his mother wasn't sure what was happening to her little boy. She knew that he was unhappy, and he demanded all of her attention. After many visits to doctors, a pediatric neurologist diagnosed his head pain as childhood migraine, which is not uncommon in families with a strong history of migraine sufferers. Armed with that diagnosis, his mother could now say to him when he rubbed his eyes and became irritable, crying and clinging: "You have a headache. You're going to lie down and let your eyes rest because they're tired. Remember what the doctor said. We'll use the special headache medicine, tuck you into your blankey, and put a nice cool cloth on your head to help the pain go away." Instead of fretting, Tyler quickly learned the ritual to relieve his pain and began to actively participate in it, because it helped him. He startled his mother one day by volunteering, "Mommy, my headache is coming back!" Tyler was no longer bewildered or helpless. He heeded his pain and took the best action possible for a four-year-old—that is, asking his parent for help.

Coping with acute pain, whether or not analgesics are used, requires one to work actively with the pain, allowing it to shift and dissipate, preventing fear from exacerbating the pain experience. When pain is continual—recurrent or chronic—it requires an even greater understanding of the nature of the pain, a greater knowledge of medications, and a repertoire of reliable coping methods. Parents who understand, interpret, comfort, and help ease the pain make it all the more bearable for children of all ages.

Every day in homes, on playgrounds, and in schoolyards throughout the world, parents and caretakers observe, assess, and interact with their children during their many childhood mishaps. Parents use pats, rub the mild bumps, and put a Band-aid on the scrape to assist the child in letting the pain go. Generally, the older the child, the less frequently the child reaches for help.

Sensitive nine-year-old Tamara landed on the top part of her foot during gymnastics. The pain was sharp and upset her intensely. Her teacher, who had first-aid training, examined her foot and said: "I can see this is hurting you lots. But as I move your toes, I don't think any of your bones are broken. That's a very good sign. I think you've bruised yourself—even though we don't see any bluish area yet, it's very tender. I'll get you an ice pack, and you sit with your foot up on this bench so that it'll ease the pain and stop any more bruising. You can watch the rest of the class, and we'll see how you feel then—okay?"

This caring teacher gave a worried, hurting child a reasonable and very plausible explanation of why her foot was causing her so much pain and suggested what to do to make it feel better. Helping to attach meaning to that pain reduced this nine-year-old's anxiety, making the pain easier to handle.

Over time, children learn to provide their own comforting rituals, such as rubbing or kissing the pain, quieting themselves in ways similar to the ways caregivers respond to younger children. The caring and comfort of parental attention—a kiss, a pat, or comforting words, such as "Now it's all over and your pain can get better"—teach children, over time, how to shift their own bodies from the shock of sudden pain or the fatigue of continuing pain to a more restful state that promotes healing and recovery.

Some parents believe that having frequent pain experiences will enable children to be less distressed by pain. This is not so. With repeated exposure children do not become less sensitive or used to pain. In fact, children who experience a lot of pain in their everyday life are often the most sensitive to pain experiences. We know that exposure to pain early in a child's life makes a child even more sensitive and preoccupied with pain. In these situations such as having a pre-term baby in the special care nursery, parents play a pivotal role in defining and mediating their child's early pain experiences by providing comfort and holding, rocking, and soothing their child. Psychologist Dr. Ruth Grunau writes: "For children who experience prolonged exposure to painful medical interventions, sensitive parenting may enhance the development of appropriate interpretations of later pain experiences, as well as coping strategies for responding to pain."

Adapting as Children Grow Older

Teenagers and some older children may reject or scorn their parent's pats or kisses, however helpful they were in the past. As Susan Lewis says in her humorous article in *Parent's Express* (1990):

Once upon a time, my kisses were magical. They could heal scraped knees and bruised egos, warm cold fingers and dampened spirits. Recently, though, they are anathema, to be avoided like ghostly slime, kryptonite, and green vegetables. "Danny," I say, looking him in the eye, "can I have one quick kiss?" He studies me as one might a slow learner. "I hate kisses." "Even from me?" "Yes." "But isn't your mom the one person who can give you a kiss now and then?" He puts his hands on my cheeks and leans towards me until our faces almost touch. His unblinking blue eyes peer into mine, and he whispers softly, "Only when I'm bleeding!" Then he stands back and grins. It is our secret. There is still some magic left.

As children grow and change, they force us to alter our ways of assisting them when they are in pain. Teenagers, for example, may demand to cope more independently with their pain and may object to having their parents' close attention. Those shifts are not always easy to make, as we are often set in our customary patterns of responding to pain. (See Chapter 4.)

If parents had the power to do so, they would organize a life that was entirely pain-free for their babies, children, and teens. Since this is beyond their control, they are left with the choice to be passive, responsive, or proactive. Whereas being passive leaves the child to make sense and manage as best as he or she can, the second two alternatives, responding to and preparing a child for coping with pain, offer the child opportunities to learn how best to manage pain and distress.

Allowing for Children's Temperamental Differences

In the challenge of responsive parenting, parents have also spoken of the need to use different coping styles with each child in the family because of temperamental differences. Children within families know their own differences. It does not appear unfair to them if a "dramatic" child is dealt with in one way, whereas the quieter, more introverted child is dealt with in another way. Children often implicitly understand their siblings' needs and differences, as long as comparisons carrying implicit judgments are not drawn between siblings.

Parents also report that they sometimes need to use different strategies at different times with the same child. This is intelligent and responsive coping, even if it is demanding for the parent. The kernel of wisdom to be extracted from studies of coping, both with adults and with children, is that how one copes is highly specific to each situation. Coping depends on the nature and intrinsic meaning of the stressful situation for each person. The same person in the same situation may cope very differently at a different time.

Methods of Coping with a Child's Pain

Since coping is a highly personal process that can vary according to the situation, how you cope when your child has a sudden onset of acute pain may be very different from how you cope when this same pain recurs two weeks later or if it should shift into a chronic pattern to which everyone in the family has to adapt. Understanding more about how you cope requires an appreciation not only of your individual coping style but also of the different stressful situations you might face when your child is in pain.

The coping process itself has four phases:

- Appraising the situation
- Encountering it
- Recovering from it
- Assessing the results of your coping.

In 1988, researchers Lazarus and Folkman investigated different types of coping strategies adults used with a particularly stressful event and arrived at eight distinct categories. They found that a person's coping skills were quite specific to particular situations and were not fixed personal patterns. Adults may use any of the following eight categories of coping to deal with stressful events.

1. *Confrontative, using aggressive efforts to alter the situation.* For example, "I stood my ground and fought for what was needed."

2. *Distancing or minimizing, downplaying the significance of the situation.* For example, "I just carried on, as if nothing had happened."

3. *Self-controlling efforts, trying to regulate feelings and actions.* For example, "I kept my feelings to myself."

4. *Use of social support, making efforts to gather information for physical or emotional support.* For example, "I called my friend who went through a similar experience for advice."

5. *Escapist or avoidant coping, including wishful thinking and efforts to escape or avoid the problem.* For example, "I tried to make myself feel better by eating [or drinking or smoking or using drugs]."

6. *Problem solving, deliberately trying to alter the situation using focused problem-solving skills.* For example, "I drew upon my past experiences and determined whether what had worked then might work now."

7. *Positive reappraisal, involving efforts to create positive meaning by focusing on personal or spiritual growth.* For example, "Going through this experience is making me change and grow as a person."

8. *Acceptance of responsibility, attempting to put it right by acknowledging one's own role in the problem.* For example, "I gave myself a lecture."

Parents draw on these coping options when dealing with a child in pain. Each can be helpful at the right time—the person under stress can judge which is best.

How a Child's Pain Affects Us

Parents and grandparents commonly feel distressed when their child or grandchild experiences pain. I have often heard them say: "This is not fair.

I wish I could have the pain so that my child didn't have to suffer," or "I wish this had happened to me rather than to my child." Sometimes a parent has admitted, after the fact: "I wanted to simply gather her up in my arms and whisk her away—away from the pain, upset, and confusion."

Some parents state categorically that the worst part of seeing their child in pain is their own sense of helplessness. When they can't do anything to take the hurt away, they feel awful. They feel dependent on others to provide that relief, which sometimes comes and sometimes does not. These feelings of dependency combined with not being able to rely on the help is distressing, frustrating, and unacceptable.

Parents tend to emotionally carry their child's pain and consequently feel overwrought, worried, or desperate unless they see evidence that adequate steps have been taken to address and ease their child's pain. Parents need to see that the pain is in fact easing and that their child is experiencing relief before their own relief can set in. The truth is that *a child in pain has a parent in pain.* The corollary to this is that *a child's pain is unfortunately also a parent's pain.*

THE NEED FOR SUPPORT

Parents work hard at managing their feelings in order to help their children through their pain. They often put their own feelings on the back burner so that their distress doesn't get in the way of giving their child love, support, and guidance to get through the distress and discomfort. Health care professionals, who are usually not involved in the extended family and the community, often do not pay attention to the cost to parents in energy, emotion, financial drain, and disruption in family and personal life when they are dealing with their suffering children. That cost is high. Parents caring for a child in pain and distress also need support and emotional outlets. The type of support is a highly personal choice, but it is necessary to have some "people of the heart" to turn to when an extra pair of ears or arms is needed. Understanding and support make it possible for parents to regain some perspective and a sense of the outside normal world or to lighten their emotional burden.

Gathering support and information from health care staff, friends, and other parents is a natural coping method. The simple act of putting your distress into words and conveying it to someone else can help you to appraise your situation and ease feelings of anger or helplessness. Parents who have gone through similar experiences with their children can provide support, strength, and the invaluable knowledge from their own experience. Parents in similar situations very quickly become allies for each other. They have something powerful in common—the pain and suffering of their children. These friendships can provide help in a way that friendships outside the current stressful situation cannot, removed as they are from these unique and demanding experiences.

COPING TECHNIQUES FOR PARENTS

Many of the methods recommended to relieve children's pain and distress can be used by parents too to ease their own tension, strain, and distress. These specific coping techniques include:

- Listening to a relaxation tape or your favorite music.
- Using imagery, visualizations, and hypnosis which, when combined with relaxation, will allow you to transform your inner experience so that you can return to your responsibilities more refreshed, with a clearer vision of your situation and its possibilities.
- Breathing deeply, which is very helpful when your energy is fading or when you become aware of accumulated body tension that needs to dissipate.
- Taking part in physical exercise, such as walking, yoga, swimming, or cycling, to relieve tension and to allow a rebalancing of your emotional and physical energies.
- Taking a soothing massage or a refreshing warm bath or shower.
- Using medication and prayer as natural ways of drawing on extra strength to continue.
- Writing letters to important people in your life or keeping a personal diary or journal. The writing process can focus, contain, and increase your own understanding of your experience with a child in pain.

Many parents have commented that keeping a journal over time to track their child's episodes of pain is a valuable coping and assessment aid. It helps identify the pain patterns and lessen the uncertainty of pain that occurs at home or in hospital. By examining the journal you can identify the early signs of pain or the factors that worsen the pain. The journal can therefore be used to advocate for better pain relief from a position of evidence and knowledge. When using a journal to better understand the pain, address these questions:

- What time of day or night does the pain occur?
- What else coincides with the pain or has preceded the onset of the pain within the last hour?

- How long does it last?
- What worsens it?
- What helps the pain settle?
- How long is your child pain-free?

The value of keeping a journal can be seen in what happened to fifteen-year-old Tamiko.

An antibiotic capsule stuck in her throat and dissolved, burning her esophagus. She was in recurrent acute pain. Her pain treatment in hospital consisted of an opioid IV infusion. Her mother was puzzled about why Tamiko had increased pain episodes during the day yet seemed much more comfortable at night. The house staff maintained that she had been given enough pain-relieving medication during the day to keep her comfortable but, according to Tamiko and her mother, during these acute pain episodes she was far from comfortable.

Her mother decided to keep a journal, noting exactly when Tamiko's pain increased. She also asked her daughter to rate her pain using a one-to-ten scale of pain and recorded her daughter's self-report of her pain. (Tools to help children rate their pain are covered chapter 5.) Through carefully documenting what was happening, a pattern emerged after two days. Tamiko's mother could see from her journal that within half an hour after a meal, which consisted of a "smoothie," or liquid food, Tamiko's pain would increase, getting progressively worse at each subsequent meal. Thus, her pain after her dinner smoothie was the worst. She requested that the staff observe Tamiko half an hour after her lunch and half an hour after dinner. It became clear to the physician that the food was irritating her esophageal burn and causing a spasm. She was immediately taken off food by mouth so that the tissue could heal uninterrupted by irritants. Her pain medication was reviewed and changed to include a muscle relaxant to reduce muscle spasm after drinking.

The journal was a relatively objective record that helped clarify Tamiko's pain, giving information that led to better control of her pain and a better treatment plan. If the physician had reacted negatively to the fact that Tamiko's mother was keeping a journal, or to the details of the journal, taking it as personal criticism of his medical care, then a change of physician would have been indicated. In the best interests of the child and parents, teamwork needs to be collaborative, open, and mutually respectful.

In contrast, this is how one father used a journal to cope privately with his own pain during his baby girl's prolonged medical treatment in hospital.

The father of desperately ill Anna kept a journal to hold himself together during the long days of his daughter's treatment for her congenitally malformed heart. In pain, he turned inward. He used the journal as a tool to try to make sense of the pain and suffering his five-month-old girl was undergoing. He would write daily, sometimes as he sat at her crib in the intensive care unit, after having held her hand for long quiet stretches. He noted how fragile human life is, how elemental parenthood is, how deeply bonded he felt to Anna, so frail with her wide dark eyes.

His journal writing, private and searching, helped him to deal with his pain as he stayed with his baby through her struggle to breathe and to hold onto life. He said that he knew his mind was only able to hold onto some of his thoughts and images, because his mind during this time was like a sieve. His pain was both emotional and physical—he spoke of the physical aching in his chest. Talking to a chosen few and writing in his journal were the only and best ways for Anna's father to express his pain.

When a Child's Pain Seems Too Much

Seeing a child suffer is emotionally draining for all involved. It can induce feelings of despair, exhaustion, anger, and fear, all of which can be temporarily immobilizing. Some parents in medical settings, as a consequence of their own previous terrifying medical procedures, or for other personal reasons, have declined to participate or to help relieve their child's distress and pain. I heard a parent turn to the nurse and say: "You can handle it better than I can; it's your job. I'm going!"

This parent was greatly distressed and traumatized by her child's pain; she needed help too. Being parachuted into the foreign world of a hospital, she understandably did not know that there are ways to help your child when medical procedures need to be done. In discussion afterward, she spoke about feeling helpless and not up to the task of helping her child manage the pain. She hadn't realized that for her child, her presence was of the utmost importance, indeed, more important than anything else.

The Importance of a Parent's Presence

However your child's pain is affecting you, it may be helpful to remember that just your presence, holding your child's hand, being caring and loving in the way you know best, is the *best* way to start supporting your child in pain. Even during their worst pain, children report that having one or both parents with them helped the most. We also know that however distressed and anxious parents feel, they are still able to help their children through difficult medical situations. Children remember what you do and say, even if they are hurting. Their sense of security is re-established, which helps them to settle, to begin coping, and not to fight the pain. Help can come in many subtle forms, and for children it starts with a known, loved presence.

Parents As Active Partners in Their Child's Pain Management

Handling pain is a continuing learning and coping process for all involved—not only for the child but for all caregivers, whether at home, in the community, in school, or in hospital. Professionals who work with children rely on parents' assessments and knowledge of their child's daily needs. Health professionals recognize that parents play a vital part in assessing the nature of the child's pain, carrying out some of the treatment, and monitoring the child's progress over time. In hospitals, nurses and physicians often ask for and listen closely to parents' observations, assessments, and recommendations. Here are some ways in which parents have contributed to creating more effective pain management for their child:

- Determining that one medication seemed more effective at relieving the child's pain than another and raising that for discussion with the caregiver.
- Insisting during a prolonged hospital stay that warm baths be included daily since they helped ease their child's pain.
- Asking for physiotherapy or using TENS (transcutaneous electrical nerve stimulation) rather than simply waiting for the pain to go away when nothing was offered for a teen's gnawing pain in an arm weakened by a stroke.
- Ensuring that the child established his bubble-blowing routine and felt supported before the lab technician drew the child's blood on a routine clinic visit.
- Keeping a journal that showed a teen's experience of breakthrough pain during the early hours of the morning and therefore requesting better pain coverage so that the teen could get an uninterrupted night's sleep.

All these recommendations made a significant difference in reducing the child's pain and suffering. All were legitimate, helpful, and supportive responses and illustrate how broad the parent's role is in helping a child manage pain and its inevitable distress.

In conclusion, in their early years, children absorb and learn from their parents and model their own behavior on their parents' behavior and attitudes. Most times the presence of parents in and of itself provides crucial help for a child during a painful episode. Since parents play such a central and guiding role with their children, it is important that parents feel equipped to understand and deal with their children's experience of pain and have their own sources of support.

CHAPTER 3

Responding to a Child's Pain

How to Respond to a Child's Pain

"Suffering children hurt us," says psychologist Dr. Joe Barber. What can we do to relieve this suffering? No matter what culture, belief system, or attitudes a child or an adult has, in order to respond effectively to a child in pain, an adult must *emphatically acknowledge the child's pain experience and support the child in dealing with the pain*. If you know a child well and have a trusting relationship, it is often easy to gain the child's confidence and cooperation. If you have to deal with a child in pain and you do not know the child, there is still a great deal you can do on the spot, in the first few moments with the child, that can turn a painful, fearful situation into a more manageable one. Remember that a child in acute or persistent pain is a child in need. Children want the pain to stop. They reach for help, and the help can come in many forms.

HELPFUL RESPONSES TO A CHILD'S PAIN

The following ten guidelines constitute what children have said and what research and clinical experience have indicated is helpful to a child in acute or persistent pain.

1. *Respond promptly to the child's pain in a caring and practical manner.* For example, in response to a child who has suffered a laceration at school, you might say, "That's a painful cut! We must run cool water over it to clean it up. The coolness of the water will soothe you—just feel. Now we'll take a look and see what happened to your hand." Or, if a child returning from school complains of a headache: "I'm sorry that your headache has come back so soon. You know the buildup of the pain will stop if you lie down immediately. Go get into bed and I'll bring you a Tylenol. "

2. *Inform the child about what is happening in his or her body.* For example: "You've tumbled to the bottom of the stairs, Ted. Your body may be hurting, and I don't want you to move yourself at all. You don't quite realize that you've hurt yourself. It may be serious, so please lie still. Your brother is calling the ambulance right now. I'm going to cover you with a blanket, because when you're in shock your body feels cold even if it's hot outside. Here you go. Concentrate now on feeling warm."

3. *Acknowledge the pain; don't minimize or deny it.* If a child has a stomach ache, you might say: "These stomach cramps are hurting you a lot. I can see that you're very uncomfortable. What do you think will help you the most right now? Would you like a hot water bottle to ease the cramps?" If the child is in hospital following surgery and is clearly uncomfortable and having a hard time settling, you could say: "Your pain is bothering you, isn't it? Your surgery is over, but I don't think you should be having this pain. I'll speak to your nurse so that you can get better relief than you have right now."

Children feel discounted and unrespected when their pain is not acknowledged—for example, during a diagnostic work-up when the practitioner's actions imply that he or she does not believe the child. As 16-year-old Jodi recalled: "On top of the pain, I then had people coming in and prodding me and not believing that I was in pain—just because I wasn't screaming like those cry-babies down the hall." She was later diagnosed with a rare neuromuscular disease.

4. *Make physical contact with the child in the way that feels best for you both.* Depending on your relationship, the age of the child, and the situation, you can hold hands, stroke the child's back or arm, or put your arms around the child to provide a sense of containment and protection. Physical contact also provides both physical and psychological relief when words are hard to find or the child is too distressed to listen.

5. *Pain isolates and isolation is frightening; if possible, remain with the child until the pain is under control.* Children do not want to be left alone to struggle on their own. Over and over children say that what counted for them the most when they were in pain was having Mom or Dad with them as they experienced the pain. Their presence makes the experience easier for both children and adolescents in a myriad of obvious and subtle ways. Even if you don't know the child, you should not abandon him or her prematurely: your caring attention and skill as a caretaker mitigates the child's fear of being left alone with the pain.

Even with teenagers, your presence counts for a lot. Older adolescents may inform caretakers or parents, "I can handle it on my own. I'm okay; I don't need you here all the time." But often it is important for the teen to have someone there at first. Dismissing parents who are no longer needed is thus a positive step, affirming growing competence and self-reliance. This effort deserves to be respected and supported from an acceptable distance; the teen will appreciate the opportunity to feel stronger and more independent.

Situations vary, so listen to what the teen wants. Sometimes a trusted adult's presence can enable a teen to handle the pain and discomfort. You understand. You can act as a buffer, interpreter, companion, and fall-back. *One caution:* Make sure that teens who want to handle the pain on their own don't cut themselves off from accepting the essential analgesic or physical treatment that will support their full recovery. For example, taking less than the recommended analgesic dose is not a sign of "being strong"; rather, it is inviting more than the necessary suffering. It is great to learn to handle it on one's own, but teens and children must be taught to use wisely what we know can make the experience shorter and easier. In such situations, adults who are not the teen's parent are often in a better position to instruct the teen; that is, they are at an acceptable emotional distance, and the teen can hear the message without the overlay of a dependency battle.

6. *Tell the child what positive steps are being taken or will be taken to deal with the pain.* You might say as you wait in a cubicle in the emergency department: "I know it seems a long time since we came into emergency. The nurse who first saw us knows that you're hurting. I guess we're not the most serious case they've got here today. That's the good news. The really good news is that she's checking with the physician to get some pain medication that will take the edge off your pain. Then we'll probably have to go for X-rays to find out what is causing your pain."

7. *Provide hope, wherever possible.* Children need to know that the pain will get better because of the steps being taken. Providing hope can spur a child on to face difficult procedures or trying times. Robbing a child of hope that things can change does not respect the need for the human spirit to hold onto the possibility that life will change and can get better. Hope can be engendered in many ways—by the words you use, the way you say them, the affection you convey, and the conviction you impart that this discomfort or distress will cease. Hope can include praying or affirming religious or spiritual beliefs and reminding yourself and the child that the pain can and will come to an end.

For a child with persistent pain recovering from a car accident in hospital, you might say: "I know you have had a hard time with the pains in your ribs and legs since the car accident last month. I bet you've been wondering whether it's ever going to end. Well, I have good news for you. The orthopedic specialist says that the pins can come out in two weeks' time. But you'll still have to be careful as you get back on your legs. The physiotherapist will help you begin walking, and within the month you'll be able to go home. To get your spirits up I brought you this calendar. Let's check off the days in red before your pins come out and the days in blue to complete the month. See, it's only four weeks. You'll be packing up your bags yourself sooner than you imagine."

8. *Instruct the child to do something to help the pain go away, such as breathing, blowing bubbles, using imagery and relaxation techniques, or listening to a favorite story. (These methods are explained in detail in chapter 6.)* When the child participates in becoming comfortable, his or her pain and distress are likely to ease. Active involvement moves the child from helplessness to active cooperation with the treatment team. A parent can say, "I know you feel tired and fed up right now, but I also remember how good you feel in the bath when you've played with your bubbles (or do deep relaxing breathing). Come, here's the wand. I'll blow first, and you count and see how many bubbles I've blown. Three? I bet you can do better! Here, blow! See how good that makes you feel as you blow out and let the scary feelings go? That helps the pain to settle too."

9. *Keep your own anxiety under control, since it may feed your child's anxiety.* Check your own breathing. If it is shallow and rapid or light, deliberately exhale to release any tension or muscular tightness and allow yourself to settle down. Keep breathing in a regulated fashion, such as counting in for three and releasing for three, until you feel yourself again.

In my experience working with children who had cancer and required regular painful bone marrow aspirations as part of their treatment, when the procedure was not going well, the tension in the treatment room would spiral and everyone would tense up, including me. Within a short time, the atmosphere could be cut with a knife. We learned to cue each other with: "Breathe!" Wry grins crossed our faces as everyone exhaled, releasing tension, and from then on we would all handle the procedure better. If we were not successful in managing our own anxiety in the tense situation, we would end up with a variety of symptoms, such as neck or back tension, a headache, or feeling wrung out at ten o'clock in the morning. The children naturally picked up our tension and inevitably did worse than if we had been relaxed and playful, coming from a position of strength. I thus learned how crucial it is to help myself if I wish to help others.

10. *Soothe your child's anxiety by remaining an attentive coach, closely supporting your child's coping skills.* Coping is a learned skill that varies from one situation to another, and encouragement and active guidance will help children cope. Supporting early coping efforts will set the stage for the development of more complex coping skills. Here is an example of how one dad coached his anxious seven-year-old son through the removal of his leg cast:

"I can't do it, Dad!" cried a weary Samuel. Uncertainty and fatigue nearly wrecked this child's first coping steps. His dad responded with soothing, consistent support: "I'm right here with you, Sam. It's okay, you're doing okay, just hold still for a short, short while. The cast is nearly off. You've held wonderfully still, and it's been very awkward. This is almost like the time you were wedged into the canoe with your legs twisted around our gear, remember? Remember how you had to just sit there so still because we didn't want to tip the canoe? No one risked moving around. It's like that time. The waves were coming and it was sitting-still time. You're doing so well right now. You'll soon be free."

UNHELPFUL RESPONSES TO A CHILD'S PAIN

Responding to a child in pain requires continuing empathy with the child's experience and an awareness of the impact of your words and manner. For all adults, witnessing a child in pain can generate not only empathy and the desire to help but many uncomfortable feelings as well, including frustration, anger, irritation, helplessness, and the desire that the pain end as soon as possible. These uncomfortable feelings can hamper you in being helpful to a person in pain. Following is a list of ways you should not respond to children in pain, since they will not help ease the pain or promote the child's coping with discomfort.

1. *Do not rob a child of hope.* It is inexcusable to rob a child —or anyone— of hope in the struggle with pain. Communicating during the experience of pain can be tricky, however. In the human interchange, there can be multiple layers of message, meaning, and sometimes miscommunication. Take this extreme but not uncommon scenario: A teenager, Tanh, returns to see his physician for the sixth time for the same pain in his limbs, a pain which interrupts his sleep. The physician has tried various treatments with little or no change in Tanh's pain. The physician's response, below, is not what Tanh needs to hear:

Physician: I'm afraid we've tried everything and I can't help you.

[A helpful remark would have been: "Even though we haven't managed to pinpoint the exact cause of your pain, we've managed to rule out the usual diseases that cause limb pain. But there are some pains that we don't yet understand; they linger on and can be very painful, even though we know they're not life-threatening. We don't yet know the best way to manage these pains."]

Tanh: You don't want to see me anymore?

[Inwardly he thinks: "He's telling me I'm a hopeless case."]

Physician: No, that's not it. I'm sorry, but I can't do anything more for you at this point. Come back and see me in three months' time.

Tanh: You mean I'm just going to have to live with it?

[Tanh needed to hear: "It's clear that this pain is still bothering you. I know serious limb pain, and your pain luckily does not indicate a serious disease. It's possible that you'll outgrow it. Let's give it three months; it should settle down by then. Meanwhile, use massage in this way, with heat if you wish, every night before bed."]

2. *Do not respond inconsistently.* Children in pain need to be consistently heard and believed. This confirmation occurs when adults or family members respond promptly and genuinely. Inconsistent responses, such as providing excessive emotional or physical responses at one time and telling the child to handle the pain on his or her own at another time are unhelpful at best and at worst will adversely affect how the child behaves when in pain.

If a child has been fussed over before but now is told that "nothing is the matter," he or she may go to extremes to prove to the parent that the pain is real and is really upsetting. The child may grimace more, cry more intensely, and become overconcerned about not having the pain acknowledged. Sometimes children develop other symptoms, such as headaches on top of the original stomach pains, which they may feel more intensely because of the perceived neglect.

Maria, a ten-year-old girl, explains how her little pain becomes embellished:

I mostly moan and say I don't feel very well. Sometimes my mom will say, "Okay, go and lie down." But sometimes she doesn't and just ignores me. Then I say it's both my head and my stomach, but it's usually only my stomach that hurts—it hurts a little bit, I think, but I will blow it up until my Mom says, "Okay, okay—you'd better stay home today!"

In my experience, parents are usually very sensitive to this shift in their child's behavior. Some parents in this situation will feel less sympathy and become less responsive to their child, saying to themselves that the child is acting this way for attention. Parents may also become irritated and feel manipulated by the child in pain, withdrawing further or responding with unhelpful annoyance, saying, for example: "I don't believe you," or "You're making such a big deal out of a little pain!"

3. *Avoid responding with irritation.* Withdrawing or responding with irritation will not encourage the child to deal effectively with pain. It is better to deal with pain directly, without any emotional overlay. If you feel that the child is becoming caught up with anxiety or embroidering the pain somewhat, you need to start by accepting the child's experience. Say in a kindly, matter-of-fact way: "I can see that you're still bothered by the pain. I'm sorry about that. What's happening?" After discussing the pain with the child, ask whether there is anything you can do to help.

You thereby hand some of the responsibility to the child to determine what would help ease the pain. By doing so, you demonstrate that you're not ignoring the pain or withdrawing when the child is in pain. You are staying, but you want the child to share in the process of feeling better.

Consider the case of six-year-old Melanie, who needed a check-up for her kidney condition. The check-up involved blood work, and Melanie worked herself into a state for the five days before having the needle. Her parents noticed that she was biting her nails, that she was leaving food on her plate, and that she was a listless and worried little girl.

"Is it going to hurt?" she asked. "It'll just last a minute and then will be over," answered her mother. But that didn't satisfy Melanie, who whimpered, "I don't want to have a needle, Mom." "There is nothing we can do about it, Mel," her mother answered, becoming irritated. "It has to be done to make sure you're well." I am well! And I hate needles!" cried Melanie. The discussion then deteriorated into an argument, with Mom unhappily defending why the needle was necessary for Melanie's continued well-being and Melanie arguing desperately to try to keep herself safe from the hurt.

How could Melanie's mom have better handled this very understandable fear of needles? She could have done two things to deflate Melanie's anticipatory fear without becoming irritated or withdrawing from her real concerns. First, she could have acknowledged her daughter's fear: "You're worrying about the needle again, Melanie? Tell me about what worries you the most." Second, she could have teamed up with her daughter to build a coping plan, such as using the non-prescription topical anesthetic cream, EMLA® [see p. 178] and bubble-blowing: "Remember how last time we saw that boy blowing bubbles and blowing his scary feelings away, before and while he had his needle? It went very well for him, didn't it? Would you like to do that? I'll make some bubbles out of dishwashing liquid and we can practice now."

With recurring or persistent pain, parents need to establish a modus operandi to avoid feeling exasperated or irritated by a child's pain, which may be exacerbated by other issues—for example, sibling rivalry. Here is an example of how one mother problem-solved with her son and established a consistent coping pattern.

Matt, a scholarly and rather serious 11-year-old boy, whose tension headaches frequently recurred, seemed to be particularly surly and sulky after school each day. He complained to his mother that his headaches were much worse after school, despite his effective use of massage and relaxation techniques at other times. Whatever his mother suggested he shot down with "It won't work." His mother found herself becoming increasingly irritated by his hostility and negativity. When asked what she could do to help him so that he could better help himself, Matt answered, "Get my sister to stop bugging me!" Matt's mother was rather taken aback at his vehemence.

In the past, she had tried to smooth over the differences between Matt and his talkative nine-year-old sister. She thought that her peace-making had been successful, but his tension-filled remark forced her to review her handling of the situation. This time she arranged with the two siblings that Matt have the sole use of his father's study for an hour after school. That way he would not be interrupted by anyone in the family. His job was to get himself comfortable and headache-free. Instead of being drawn into yet another sibling conflict or challenging Matt on the authenticity of his headaches, this mother listened and, after discussion with both children, provided Matt with transition time to settle himself after the rigors of school in a quiet space. This was all that Matt needed to reduce the frequency of his headaches.

4. *Don't fuss too much over the child.* What is fussing? It is doing things that are not constructive and do not provide solutions, such as asking a lot of unimportant questions to reassure yourself and not the child and physically doing things that are not essential to lessen your own anxiety, not the child's: "Oh, my poor child, what can I do? Would you like me to fluff up your pillow? Is the pain still so terrible? Oh dear, what are we going to do?" When someone is fussing, the real needs of the person in pain often become secondary or incidental. Fussing is often a reflection of feeling helpless and unsure of how to be useful.

The effect of a caretaker's or a parent's fussing over a child's mild or short-term pain episode is to send the message to the child that this is very bad pain, that the child should be alarmed by the pain and stay alert to the pain signals. The child then learns to remain sensitive to the pain signals and continues to feel the pain and be distressed. Fussing over pain weakens the child's ability to learn to cope and to draw maximum benefit from analgesics and pain-relieving strategies.

Parents who are fussing can get so emotionally overwrought that they don't pick up their children's cues that the pain is settling and they feel better now. Sometimes even when children actually push their fussing parents away by saying, "Stop it" or "Leave me alone," the preoccupied parent has difficulty taking in the message. The more stoic child or adolescent may respond to fussing with irritation: "I can handle it. It's okay, don't fuss. Get off my back!" Meanwhile, he or she may be a long way from truly being on top of the pain.

In the family's life, the impact of a parent's fussing or asking too many questions places too great a focus on the child's pain. Over time, the child learns that his or her pain has power in the family, that it can worry Dad and Mom and take attention away from brothers and sisters. It can get people to do things that they wouldn't usually do. This power may scare the child. Some children in pain have reported wondering, in the extreme of their pain and the family's distress, if their pain was life-threatening. They think, "Mom and Dad have never behaved like this before; maybe my condition is a lot more serious than I thought. Maybe I'm going to die." An overfocus on the child's pain can therefore change family dynamics.

Bright, 12-year-old Kate had stomach pains. Her pediatrician initially diagnosed a gastrointestinal virus with accompanying diarrhea. A month later, the diarrhea had stopped, for the virus was dormant or out of her system, but her pain persisted in a vague, almost habitual way. Her mother said that Kate had become the focus of parental concern at the expense of the other two children. Her pain had changed the family dynamics.

How had that happened? Kate had become miserable and whiny and would say, "I'm never going to get better. You know, 12-year-old kids can die!" Her parents were very worried and continually asked her how she was. Her mother would drive many miles to the other side of town to buy her special yogurt. After a month of these trips she wanted to stop, but Kate continued to complain of stomach pain and refused to return to school, trapping herself and her family in despair. They all needed help and agreed to go for family therapy. After four sessions, two with the family and two by herself, Kate began to shift away from the "sick role." She started to develop some confidence and independence by learning self-regulatory techniques to "let the pain go," and her parents were freed from the unproductive patterns of fussing.

How much attention is enough? How much is too much? You will quickly notice when your child feels better and is ready to resume activities. For mild recurring pains, stay with practical solutions. If the child's pain does not respond to these solutions, or if there are troubling pains that seem out of the ordinary or won't settle, consult your physician. Also ask your child or teen for an opinion. Children of all ages are capable of telling us if this pain seems different, if it is more serious, or if it is something that will settle. Ask the child what she needs or knows to be helpful in getting the pain under control. The pain is in the child's body. Let her guide you in helping her to feel better and in making her life as normal as possible.

5. *Don't ignore the child's pain.* People who are not closely attached to the child or teen are more likely to minimize or deny the child's pain than are parents. Staff who work a lot with pain can be either very sensitive to the signs and experience of pain or emotionally distant from the child's pain.

I first witnessed someone ignoring a child's pain during an eight-year-old boy's bone marrow aspiration—a very painful ten-minute invasive procedure in which a needle is bored into the hip bone to extract a sample of marrow. The boy was doing his best, attempting to relax, but the local anesthetic clearly was not enough. He was feeling the pain and cried out, "It's hurting!" The physician, a skilled but very cool, controlled, and dispassionate woman, said with her voice of authority, "It's not hurting!" With shock, the rest of us almost in one voice said, "But he says it is hurting—so he needs more local anesthetic!" Suffice it to say, there was a battle of words that would not have occurred if the physician had not been emotionally distant and out of touch with the child and had not denied the pain the child was feeling.

Certainly some parents, distressed when their child is in pain, cope by denying or minimizing their child's pain. Over the years they build up a protective wall to keep themselves from experiencing these uncomfortable feelings. One response is to downplay their child's pain, to ignore it, or to leave the child to manage—perhaps in the way that the parent was treated as a child. In these instances, the child does not recognize that his mom or dad is acting out of self-protection. The child learns that pain is something you have to handle on your own. So he too builds a wall of protection, carrying a lot of tension in his body and rarely asking for emotional or physical support or for medication during the pain.

Sometimes in this stoic reaction, the child does quietly draw on internal resources and images and learns spontaneously to dissociate himself from the pain. Twelve-year-old Kevin was one of these inwardly resourceful youngsters. He had to have a number of myelograms that required spinal taps. His parents didn't think it was "a big deal," and Kevin did not ask his mother to accompany him. He told us that "I just make myself relax, like I'm a wet noodle!" Imagining him as a limp noodle resting warmly in a bowl of noodles is one of my favorite spontaneous images of all time! Needless to say, Kevin coped remarkably well.

Downplaying a child's pain may unfortunately be a sex-biased phenomenon. Researchers Fearon and McGrath noted in a study of everyday pain among young children that young girls receive physical comfort twice as often as young boys, that girls receive physical comfort whenever the caregiver is nearby and is aware of a pain incident, without being prompted by the child's sobs, cries, or screams. In contrast, boys receive physical comfort only when they are in tears. With these findings in mind, we need to monitor how we respond to young boys, since our responses could have long-range effects on their sense of support during pain and on their right to express their feelings when they are in pain.

6. *Don't use the myth of two pains.* Parents of children with puzzling kinds of pain, such as recurring abdominal, headache, or limb pains that don't fit neatly into a recognizable syndrome and do not appear related to disease or trauma, often struggle to gain help and a clear idea of what is happening to their child. Unfortunately, at clinics and during hospital visits they encounter remarks that are at best unhelpful and at worst reveal a poor appreciation of the complexity of pain pathways.

The following unhelpful remark expressed a common variation on the myth of two pains and also dismissed the child's pain: "Since we can find no organic cause for the pain, it must be psychological" (as if pain in the body does not involve the brain). A helpful remark would have been: "Our tests have excluded any known disease that may be causing your child's pain. But we know that pain can be caused not only by disease in an organ but by more complex factors involving the brain and giving rise to pain in that organ. In these instances, other methods, such as psychotherapy or play therapy, that address the child's feelings, fears, and fantasies are needed to give him relief from the pain."

Children and teens are very sensitive to the messages associated with their conditions.

Fifteen-year-old Crystal had made two emergency room visits to the local children's hospital, throwing up and experiencing acute abdominal pains. When the hospital staff could find no clear organic cause, she said: "I felt a failure and I was confused. Maybe it was in my head; maybe I was making it all up? But it hurt so much I didn't know what to do! So they put me through all these tests, and they all came up negative. Now I really felt awful. Maybe they thought I was making it all up!" What Crystal needed was validation that, although it was difficult to identify exactly what was causing her pain, it was clear to all that she was in pain, and that she would not be cast aside just because her pain did not fit neatly into an easy diagnostic category.

Sometimes, if children do not feel heard or supported in their pain and distress, they become angry. They can end up not trusting the very people they have come to for help. (As 11-year-old Bryan, who had irritable bowel syndrome), said: "When I could see that the doctor did not believe my pain, I felt so alone. No one could help me! It was no use." As a result of his accumulated anger and disappointing early encounters with the health care team, Bryan did not come regularly for his sessions, making it difficult for any of his professional helpers to develop a pain therapy program. His interrupted medical and psychological therapy became drawn out and ineffective. We must prevent children from losing the trust that they will receive help. The consequences of this breach are anger, rage, despair, and a legacy of inadequately treated pain.

7. *Avoid overusing sympathy.* This is a case of a caring parent who responded to his child's pain with lots of sympathy but provided no guiding information or encouragement for coping or allowing the pain and distress to settle. Four-year-old Hailey was playing in her father's office. She pinched her finger in a three-ring binder as it was closing and shrieked with shock.

Hailey: Waaaaaaaa!!!

Dad: Oh! It's bleeding! It must be very sore.

Hailey: (Crying intensifies after observing her dad's startled expression and hearing that the bleeding finger must be very sore.)

Dad: We'll have to get a Band-aid when we get home. (There is none in the office and home is 20 minutes away.)

Hailey: (Continues to cry intensely. She is preoccupied with the blood on her finger and stares fixedly at it through her sobbing.)

Dad: I'm sure it hurts a lot.

The sympathy that this supportive parent provided escalated the child's absorption in the pain. His concern promoted her belief that some terrible injury had occurred to her finger. In fact, she did not let up her intense sobbing until they reached home 25 minutes later and the Band-aid was on her finger! The Band-aid had marvelous pain-relieving properties: it worked immediately.

Hailey's father could have responded more effectively, however. Running cold water over her finger in the washroom (every office has one) would have eased the pain and washed the blood away. Her finger could have been wrapped in a clean handkerchief or tissue, and she could have been told that this would help it to feel better. When the child cannot see the blood and the injury is covered, it doesn't hurt as much. Hailey also could have been told to blow on her wrapped finger to ease the pain. It is impossible to cry and blow at the same time, and her regulated blowing would have eased her tension and distress. She would have felt better doing something to help herself, apart from crying—which, given a choice, most children would rather not do. She also needed to be told that the sharp pain helped her to get her finger out of the way of the rings, and now that her finger was safe, the pain would soon go away.

Parents As Protectors versus Restrainers

Parents are their child's protectors. The parents' need to protect the child from pain, however, can clash with the child's need for painful medical treatments. It is striking, nevertheless, how many young children are clearly able to appreciate that their parent is not an accomplice in causing the pain, particularly when they experience their parent as supportive, caring, and in continual contact.

Take, for instance, the unsettling issue of holding a child still for a procedure that involves some degree of discomfort. Providing children with the opportunity to remain still without being held is always preferable: those who are successful will achieve a sense of mastery, and those who cannot manage to stay still then understand why they must be held. There are situations, such as a physician's brief examination of a painful ear, where it is obviously necessary that a parent hold a child firmly for half a minute, particularly if a toddler or young child is feverish and cannot hold still. In the hospital, however, where a painful medical procedure requiring a young child to be still will take longer than a minute, it is not in the child's or the parents' best interests for parents to hold, subdue, or restrain their own child. For most children new to hospital, being held still by their parents against their will is confusing, even infuriating. Being asked to restrain their child for medical procedures therefore places parents in a very difficult situation; in helping the staff, they risk antagonizing their child and betraying the child's trust.

In summary, except for a short examination or immunizations, parents should not be asked to participate in restraining and holding their child down for a painful exam. It is the medical and nursing staff's job to gain the most cooperation from the child, to explain, negotiate, bargain, or, in the final extreme of medical necessity, use acceptable forms of restraint. The parent should not confuse roles by holding down a child against his or her will. The parent's job is to be there, to support and comfort the child, and to be a safe haven after the painful exam or procedure is over.

Even when parents are not asked to restrain their child, they may fear being with their child during a painful medical procedure, since they cannot provide protection from the pain. During her daughter's painful medical treatment, Chelsey's mother offered this reasoning: "If I go in there with Chelsey during her spinal tap, she'll see me as one of the bad guys hurting her. I don't want to risk that!" She feared that her presence during a painful procedure would break the trust she had with her daughter. Chelsey was three years old, but even at that age she was able to tell the difference between the role of a mother who knows and loves her and that of the hospital staff doing the procedure.

After Chelsey's mother and I discussed her fears, she blurted out with intensity: "I can't stand all these things being done to my child!" It became clear that Chelsey's mother was struggling with her powerful feelings of anger, distress, and ambivalence about the invasive and painful medical procedures that her child had to undergo as part of her medical treatment. These strong emotions had got in the way of her establishing a role for herself in the treatment as Chelsey's mother—the authority on and best help for her daughter. Her anger had so immobilized her that she could not help Chelsey.

After talking it out, this mother was soon able to begin to let go of her anger and be more helpful when Chelsey was in pain. Two weeks later she had worked out with Chelsey that she would come into the treatment room, stroke her head during her spinal tap, and cuddle her when it was all over. The impact on Chelsey was remarkable. She settled quickly after the spinal taps, and her mother felt affirmed in her ability to love and do the best for her daughter, even when she was in pain.

Children are usually very attuned to their parents' emotional state and can feel Mom or Dad's distress that something painful has to be done in the name of treating their condition. Appreciating the dilemma that their parents are in, children rarely take out their rage against them. Never have I heard a child say, "You're not a good parent because you let the doctor hurt me," even though children understandably feel very angry at being sick and having painful medical treatments.

When Your Child Is Angry at You

If the child has not been given adequate preparation or adequate pain medication and the procedure hurts, the child's anger can raise her level of distress. When, in the child's eyes, the only "acceptable" target for her anger is a parent, how should the parent handle this? Remember what the child is really angry about. Anger in these situations is a fundamental protective reaction: to defend himself or herself and stop the hurt. It is crucial that the child's anger not be taken as a personal attack. Anger is the child's natural defense. If your child lashes out, put that understanding into words and protect yourself physically.

For example, when seven-year-old Juan lashed out at his mother, she said: "Juan, I know you're mad as anything that the needle hurt. I'm so sorry that it did. But hurting me, punching me, isn't going to take the hurt away. Stop! Don't hit me! It's not okay. Are you mad at me for letting them give you a needle? We needed a sample of your blood to find out why you've been feeling so ill. It will tell us if you have a virus or some bacteria. Listen: Would you like to see what your blood looks like under a microscope?" A little intense diversion is always a good strategy, particularly if it helps the child learn more about his body!

Children also become angry if they're not told about a procedure that lies ahead, or the pain of an intervention is downplayed in the mistaken belief that it will decrease the child's anxiety. The rationale for this may be: If we don't talk about it, it will not be so bad. This strategy does not work. In fact, the child may feel justifiably angry and betrayed, struggling in isolation to make sense of the experience.

Of course, it is preferable that you not reach the point where the child's distress and anger are directed toward you and others involved in the treatment. To that end, ensure before the procedure or treatment that your child has some understanding of the situation. Preparing your child for pain as best as you can means providing as much accurate sensory and procedural information as your child can handle. Discuss with the nurse or doctor whether there is a plan, what the procedural steps are, and what your child can expect and will feel so that there are no surprises. You are then in a position to ensure that your child, no matter what age, understands the following:

- What is wrong with his body right now;
- What needs to happen for him to get well again;
- Why the health professional is doing the procedure;
- What it is called and how it could feel;
- What he can do to best help himself get through it; and
- What he could ask you, his support person, to do.

In conclusion, when children experience their parents as supportive, caring, and in close contact, they appreciate that their parents are not accomplices in causing any pain that arises from their disease, injury, or medical intervention. Parents can help their child cope through discussion, explanation of what is happening, planning, and flexible teamwork as the pain situation unfolds and different steps are taken.

CHAPTER 4

How Pain Works

When you understand how pain works, it is easier to deal with a painful experience and to make appropriate decisions on your own or with nursing and medical staff. If you explain to children and teenagers why they are hurting and how a proposed method will control their pain, they too will be better able to handle the experience.

The Pain System at Work

In every pain experience the brain integrates sensory and emotional information as well as thought processes. The following four scenarios illustrate the importance of the context in which pain occurs to define the meaning, and therefore the experience, of a pain signal.

Scenario 1: While working in your workroom, you stub your toe and feel a sudden sharp pain. You see the table leg and think, "Oh, that is what hurt my toe. It's just a stubbed toe. I've had this pain before, and even though it's killing me right now, it will settle down in a while." Because you found the reason for your pain, have placed it in context, and feel reassured about the pain, you activate an inhibitory pain system that originates in your brain and exerts control over nerve circuitry in the spinal cord. Recognizing that this pain is minor, the brain releases neurotransmitters, hormones, and other chemical substances down the spinal cord, gradually spreading pain relief.

Scenario 2: You are moving around the same workroom and feel the exact same sharp pain in your toe, but you can't see or think of anything to account for the sudden pain. You begin to worry: "What on earth is going on with my big toe?" You retrieve any earlier toe-pain experiences that you may have had and any information that could explain the sharp pain. With no explanations and mounting anxiety, you will probably feel the painful sensation more acutely. Suddenly you remember your physician's words: "The pain of a broken bone is so intense that there is no doubting that something serious is going on!" "Oh," you think, "maybe my toe is broken!" Feelings of alarm or fear increase sensitivity to the pain sensations. This pain is experienced quite differently from the toe pain described in scenario 1, where the reason for the pain was apparent. In this instance, your brain remains vigilant, trying to determine whether your toe is indeed broken and whether the pain is spreading to other parts of your body, and you will probably remain attentive to those signals until treatment is well under way.

Scenario 3: You are joking around with a good friend. Your play becomes physical, and your buddy slaps your shoulder in jest. How would the pain of that slap feel? Probably no big deal, since it is part of the horseplay. You are fond of your buddy, and you play down any discomfort.

Scenario 4: Someone you know but are somewhat afraid of is talking with you and slaps your shoulder. How different that slap feels. It may have no more intensity than the playful slap, but it takes on a radically different meaning: insult, intimidation, or possibly the threat of abuse. You may feel outraged, frightened. As an experience of pain, it is very likely that you hardly felt the playful slap in scenario 3 and easily dismissed it as "goofing around," whereas this slap may smart for a long time and may become the basis for further action.

Our central nervous system is a dynamic, continual feedback system in which our sensations, perceptions, emotions, and reactions constantly interact. As a result, what begins as a potentially painful message in one part of the body may not necessarily be transmitted to the brain and interpreted as an equally strong pain message. When brain and body rapidly develop in childhood, the nervous system is even more sensitive to influences from within the body, other people, the environment, memories, and learning. Thus, pain can have an even greater impact on a child's changing nervous system.

Unfortunately, because outdated notions persist, this interweaving of influences on the experience of pain has often been neglected. Many societies have integrated body-mind beliefs and practices. Our western culture, however, has a long tradition of ignoring the influence of the brain on the experience of pain. Despite earlier medical literature that suggested that the cerebral cortex, where the highest level of pain processing takes place, is not necessary for the experience of pain, we now know that ultimately all pain is experienced in the brain; and given the importance of learning, memories, and emotions in the experience of pain, the cerebral cortex has to be involved.

THE PROCESSING OF PAIN

When the body experiences an injury, nerve impulses at the site of the injury send a message to the brain. The nerve impulses alone are not the pain; only when they reach the brain are they defined, felt, and experienced as "pain." (For convenience, terms such as "pain message" or "pain pathways" are used in the following discussion to describe the nerve impulse; bear in mind, however, that until this impulse reaches the brain, it is just that—an impulse, devoid of meaning.) Without becoming caught up in too many Latin or Greek names, or physiological complexities, here are the broad outlines of how pain is processed in our nervous system.

Figure 4.4 shows how a nerve impulse from an injury to the toe travels up the spinal cord, reaching the brain stem and the cerebral cortex. When an injury occurs in a toe, the nerve impulses signaling the presence of an injury are rapidly transmitted as a chain reaction of electrochemical messages into the dorsal horn of the spinal cord and up the spinal cord to the brain stem. At the brain stem, the nerve impulses of the injury are relayed through the thalamus, a complex central integrating and relay center, and are routed to all parts of the cerebral cortex, including those associated with memory, cognition, emotion, and sensation. The impulses are rapidly processed by the cerebral cortex, which draws on previous experiences, current feelings, mood, the context, and the meaning the person ascribes to that unpleasant sensation.

The brain decides if what is being experienced is "pain" and how to deal with it. If alarmed by the nerve impulses, the system speeds up the transmission and intensity of the pain. If the brain determines that the pain is tolerable and not alarming, however, a descending inhibitory control system is activated. Natural body-based pain-relieving substances (endorphins—endogenous morphinelike substances) are released by the brain through the spinal cord and, together with other modulating substances, such as serotonin and norepinephrine, ease the experience of pain.

WHAT HAPPENS WHEN NERVES "TALK" TO EACH OTHER?

Information about changes in our body is transmitted by nerves in the peripheral nervous system, which consists of all the nerve fibers throughout the body that carry information to the spinal cord and the brain. The nerve fibers in the spinal cord and the brain are known as the central nervous system. Two kinds of nerve fibers transmit messages

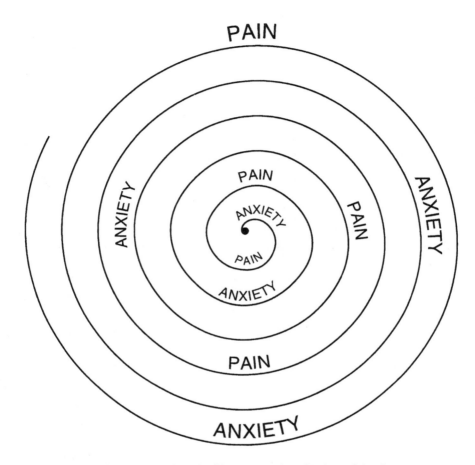

Figure 4.1 *The Spiralling Interaction of Pain and Anxiety*

about injury or tissue changes: C fibers, which are small and transmit sensation slowly, and A delta fibers, which are large and transmit sensation rapidly. C fibers transmit messages slowly because they are unmyelinated; myelin is a thin layer of protein that wraps around the nerve fibers and accelerates the speed of nerve impulse transmission.

Although both A delta and C fibers relay messages from heat, chemical, or mechanical stimulation, they produce different qualities of pain. Remember the earlier example of the stubbed toe? The immediate sharp, stinging pain in the toe was produced by the more rapidly acti-

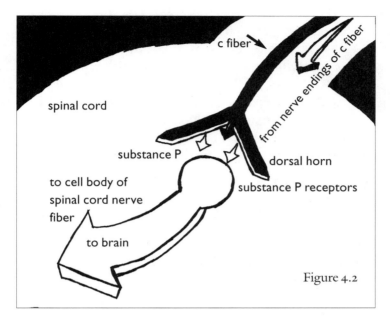

Figure 4.2

vated A delta fibers. A second or two later, the smaller and more slowly conducting C fibers produced a burning, more diffuse pain sensation that tended to outlast the initial stinging pain. It is essential that we have both of those types of pain fibers. If we didn't have the A delta fibers, for instance, the first sharp pain may not have been felt and we might not have quickly moved our toe away from the table leg to prevent further injury.

The pain message is carried along the C and A delta fibers and relays the message to the nerves at the spinal cord. When one nerve fiber, such as a C fiber, converses with a neighboring nerve cell in the spinal cord, special chemicals known as neurotransmitters are released from the first cell to the neighbor (see *figure 4.2*). According to current research, the most important pain neurotransmitter is the peptide substance P, which stands not for *pain*, but for the *powder* in which it was isolated. Researchers in the last 30 years have found not only that some of the C fibers synthesize substance P but also that it is carried into the spinal cord, where it is stored, ready to be released when "pain" messages are activated.

Substance P, released following injury, can spread over large distances in the spinal cord, exciting those cells that transmit the injury message to the brain. It comes closest to being the "pain" transmitter in the body. This wide release can also explain why some pains are difficult to localize and why some injuries often result in an achy sensation over a large region of the body, persisting longer than expected.

As researchers understand more about pain transmission at the spinal cord level, more possibilities for blocking the passage of the pain signal up to the brain are emerging. Researchers are synthesizing drugs that block the "pain-producing" action of substance P, as well as exploring substances that can cross the blood-brain barrier, to help in the treatment of migraine and other pain conditions.

HOW THE PAIN SIGNAL TRAVELS UP THE SPINAL CORD TO THE BRAIN STEM

The message of pain follows two pathways to the brain stem and it appears that these two systems transmit different types of pain information. Sharp or acute pain travels up the spinothalamic pathway to the thalamus, whereas achy pain, which is often more diffuse and difficult to localize in the body, is probably carried by the reticular formation in the brain stem. As the pain message reaches the higher brain centers, it combines with other information in the brain, including messages that underlie our thoughts, feelings, memories, and specific sensory characteristics, such as smell, sight, and sound. The brain integrates all of these features, which contribute to the final pain experience.

Puzzles in the Pain Process

There are some puzzles in the processing of pain messages. With our growing understanding of pain, some of these puzzles can now be explained, but others remain puzzling, reminding us of the intricacy and complexity of the pain process.

WHY DON'T WE EXPERIENCE THE SAME PAIN EVERY TIME FROM THE SAME INJURY?

One might think that a large injury should always result in a large amount of pain. In fact, this is not necessarily true, because the pain message can be altered in many areas within the pain pathway from the source of the pain to the brain (which will be discussed in the next sections on pain control). Many variables influence the quality and intensity of the pain experience. Clinicians and parents have noted that the same child experiencing the same type of pain within the same time frame on a subsequent occasion may experience it very differently. The meaning and context of the pain for the child can vary, affecting and in-

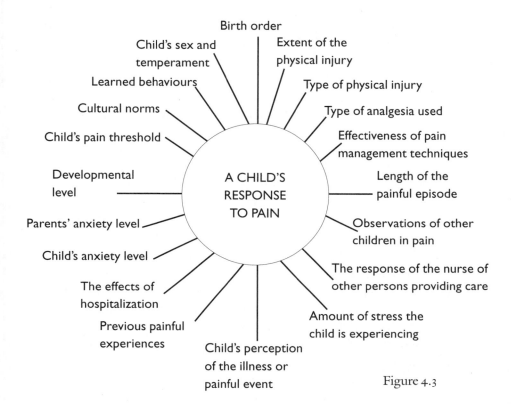

Figure 4.3

teracting with the physiologic release of chemical substances. In fact, our pain systems are not fixed or rigid but are highly plastic. Thus, we may respond differently to the same pain stimulus, depending on a multitude of factors (see *figure 4.3*), including cultural attitudes and subtle changes of context, mood, energy, and anxiety levels.

HOW DOES PERSISTENT PAIN DIFFER FROM ACUTE PAIN?

Another piece of the pain puzzle is how the various nerve fibers interact with each other and change as a result of injury. Nerve fibers themselves are damaged when the body suffers injury or amputation. In addition, their moderating influence on the C fibers decreases or is lost. When nerve fibers are injured, they no longer behave normally, as they do in an acute pain situation, but become easily irritated. Often the fibers spontaneously send impulses and are not able to stop. The pain signals can be very insistent and troubling. The brain may interpret the increased C fiber activity as arising from severe injury, and the person will then feel greater pain.

Pain due to injury to nerves (neuropathic pain) has a burning quality. This pain is no longer protective or helpful; it has become persistent and perhaps chronic. The nervous system has changed, specific nerve fibers have become irritated and more sensitive, and the person in pain requires skilled, individualized treatment programs to provide enduring relief. Pain that persists is more difficult to live with and to treat than acute pain, which lasts only a short time. For a successful outcome, the thinking, feeling, and behavior of the child and the support of other people become pivotal components of the medical treatment of persistent pain.

WHY IS PAIN IN ONE AREA FELT IN ANOTHER AREA?

Pain isn't always what it appears to be. The complex pain system has a curious manifestation known as "referred" pain. Angina, for example, can be experienced as referred pain in one part of the body, such as the shoulder or arm, even though the injury is in a deeper internal structure, the heart. During a heart attack, the pain is commonly referred from the heart to the shoulder because of the converging impulses sent into the spinal cord from both internal organs and other parts of the body. It is thought that the brain attributes the information to the more familiar part of the body for sensory messages, the shoulder or arm, thus incorrectly locating the source of the pain.

Another example of referred pain is appendicitis pain. The beginning pain of an acutely inflamed appendix, which is located in the lower right quadrant of the belly, can be first experienced as diffuse pain around the belly button and not pain in the location of the appendix. As the inflammation increases, the pain characteristically spreads and moves down to include the lower right quadrant of the abdomen. It is well known that the brain, which often cannot accurately perceive the origin of these pains, ascribes the pain to the skin or to a part of the body that is closer to the surface, where pain is more commonly experienced. Presented in this way, a child's pain may initially be confusing and yet reminds us again of the complexity of the pain experience.

WHY DO MUSCLES SOMETIMES BECOME PAINFUL WITHOUT EXPERIENCING DIRECT INJURY?

Pain can also affect muscles and ligaments. This condition is called myofascial pain, which is pain in the thin covering of the muscle. It can be manifested in different ways, such as tension headaches or achy pain in the muscles of the limbs, called fibromyalgia. For reasons that are not fully understood, the muscles become tight and painful, developing ar-

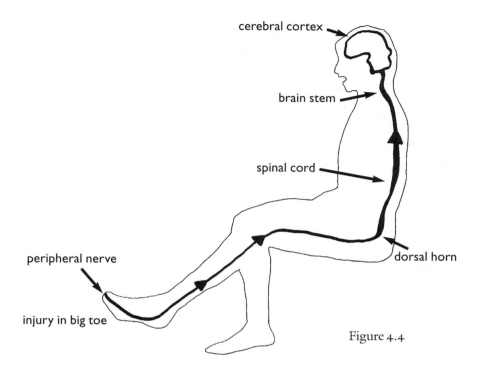

cerebral cortex

brain stem

spinal cord

peripheral nerve

dorsal horn

injury in big toe

Figure 4.4

The cerebral cortex, brain stem, and spinal cord make up the central nervous system.

eas called trigger points. These points trigger or radiate the pain into another point of the body, especially when the muscle is used or the trigger points are pressed.

Fibromyalgia is one such condition of muscle pain; this syndrome is seen primarily in adults and teenagers—girls in particular. Certain areas of the muscles over the entire body become exquisitely tender and sensitive to touch. In the absence of other musculoskeletal disease, a certain number of these trigger points in predictable parts of the body are used in diagnosing fibromyalgia.

Someone suffering from chronic daily headaches may have muscles constantly in spasm from poor posture, overuse of the muscles, or chronic stress. The neck muscles develop trigger points that are intensely painful when pressed, and the pain radiates from that point to the head, perpetuating the pain. A cycle of pain and muscle spasms then develops: a trigger causes a muscle to spasm, irritating the associated nerve, which then irritates the muscle. Once set in motion, the cycle escalates the pain.

One kind of pain can even cause another kind of pain. For example, when a bone is fractured, muscles contract, and the contracted muscles themselves also become a source of pain on top of the original pain of the fractured bone. In addition, chronically painful muscles may cause changes in posture and spasms of surrounding muscle groups, spreading the pain. Known as secondary pains, these can be very distressing and can become as much of a problem as the original pain. Aids such as physical therapy, relaxation techniques, TENS (transcutaneous electrical nerve stimulation), ultrasound, medication, and improvements in dealing with stress are helpful and necessary to break the cycle, which would otherwise persist.

HOW DOES INJURY CAUSE A "MEMORY" OF PAIN?

When an injury persists and the pain is not effectively blocked or reduced, long-term changes in the nervous system and "memory" for pain in the spinal cord occur. A recent and fascinating breakthrough has been the discovery of genes that are "turned on" by painful stimulation. The activity of genes that synthesize and regulate the neurotransmitters dramatically increases as a result of painful stimulation. We should therefore not think of the "pain" transmission pathway as a telephone cable that merely sends information from one place to the next. Neurobiologist Dr. Allan Basbaum suggests we think of it as a voice mail system:

When a "pain" message enters the central nervous system, it can be stored for long periods of time. The molecular changes that occur establish a memory trace of the injury. The memory of the injury can influence the subsequent transmission of information along this pathway.

This recent finding provides yet another reason for treating and controlling the pain of children *as soon as possible.*

WHY IS SURGERY NOT NECESSARILY
THE BEST INTERVENTION FOR PERSISTENT PAIN?

The discovery that the body can "remember" pain throws more light on why surgical interventions for relief of chronic pain have only limited success. It used to be thought that simply cutting these fibers, as one would a telephone wire that carries the pain message to the brain, would provide pain relief. We now know that cutting the fibers rarely relieves pain, or does so only transiently; indeed, surgical intervention can cause more pain. A useful analogy is that of an unplugged or cut telephone cord. Even if the electrical current can travel only to the severed point, the current is still present and running and the signals may become jangled and not be properly interpreted. Unlike a telephone wire, the body tries to heal the severed nerve portions of the peripheral nervous system, sometimes causing more pain. Damage to the central nervous system, however, is irreversible: the nerves that have been cut in the brain and the spinal cord never regenerate normal connections. Consequently, surgical interventions for chronic pain, in particular, are now infrequently performed, and techniques that do not destroy nerve tissue have been developed.

HOW DO SOME SYNDROMES
INCREASE SENSITIVITY TO PAIN?

Certain syndromes, often initiated through injury or diseases, such as rheumatoid arthritis and reflex sympathetic dystrophy, dramatically increase sensitivity to pain. In addition, injured or inflamed body tissue releases chemical substances, such as prostaglandins, that act on nerve endings, lowering their "pain" threshold. They sensitize the small C fibers, and so previously non-painful stimuli can now produce burning, achy, dull, or diffuse persistent pain. The pain of sunburn is a common example of sensitization. The lightest touch or slightest movement can be experienced as excruciatingly painful on sunburned skin. Even a warm shower is felt as a hot, painful shower, because the nerve endings in the sunburned skin have become highly sensitive.

In reflex sympathetic dystrophy, for instance, sensations that might not have previously caused the child pain, such as gently touching the skin with a cotton ball, can now produce pain. The brain interprets the sensation signals as if they were injury signals, and therefore the child experiences pain, even though the touch of a cotton ball on skin is clearly not an injury sensation. The pain system itself becomes the problem by producing extreme sensitivity. This sensitivity is known as hyperalgesia.

HOW CAN PAIN LAST WHEN
THE PAINFUL SITE NO LONGER EXISTS?

Sometimes practitioners cannot find a reason for pain in the body and conclude that it is not "real" pain, despite the patient's evident distress and reports to the contrary. Phantom limb pain exemplifies the fallacy that pain has to be located to be real. Phantom pain is not physically located. Twenty percent of children and adults experience pain in the absent limb after it is amputated as a result of an injury or disease. Children will report sharp, throbbing pain or itching in a limb that is no longer there. It is evident that the child is in pain and suffering, yet the source of the pain, the injured limb, had been surgically removed, a day or even weeks or months before.

The child knows the limb is gone, but the child's brain, perhaps interpreting the pain signals within the familiar brain neurological mappings as body pain sensations, has not yet adjusted to the radical change and loss of sensation in that limb. Although the neurological mechanisms of phantom pain are still poorly understood, our current understanding is that the brain remains "open" to the sensation that used to be received. If the child had severe pain before amputation, which is common, it is more likely that he or she will experience phantom pain after surgery. It seems that the brain and nerve pathways were sensitized to those sensations. Pain sensation over time changed the nerve fibers and cells of the stump, spinal cord, and brain, increasing the sensitivity to pain. With treatment, and over time, this pain tends to diminish, and eventually disappears.

Phantom pain exemplifies the complexity of the pain experience and the challenges of providing sound pain management. Sometimes an epidural block is given before, during, and after amputation: the nerves of the limb that are to be amputated are blocked with local anesthetic so that the injury messages produced by the surgical amputation do not reach the spinal cord. In this strategy, also called a pre-emptive block, analgesics or local anesthetics are injected into the epidural space surrounding the spinal cord up to 72 hours before surgery to block a segment of body sensation at the specific area where the pain is experienced. This analgesic technique is believed to pre-empt and block the increase in post-operative pain that will occur with surgery and to reduce the pain in the injured area, as well as to pre-empt some of the body's response to surgical amputation. The pre-emptive analgesic block appears to decrease the likelihood that phantom pain will occur. This phenomenon has fascinated many researchers, who are currently attempting to understand and to prevent this traumatic pain experience.

Pain Control

Pain can be physiologically controlled within the body in a number of ways. What begins as a potentially strong message in one part of the body is not necessarily transmitted to the brain and interpreted as a strong pain message. This section explores what is known about brain-body pain control systems.

During this century, the pain network of nerve fiber pathways into and along the spinal cord to the brain stem and brain, as well as the descending control from the brain to the spinal cord, have been extensively researched. One of the most celebrated pain researchers is Canadian physiological psychologist Dr. Ronald Melzack, whose 1973 book *The Puzzle of Pain* is now a classic. Some of the methods of controlling pain within the body that are discussed in his book are summarized below.

GATING THE PAIN

A pain signal goes through various physiological "gates," which either increase or decrease the amount of information about the pain that is transmitted along the pain pathways. These gates recur at many sites, from the source of the pain all the way to the brain, thus allowing the pain to be "gated," or regulated, at any of these sites. Some examples of gating along the pain pathway follow.

Gating in the spinal cord

As nerve fibers enter the spinal cord, they converge. The spinal nerve cells thus respond to *both* painful and non-painful stimulation, because they receive input both from large touch, and movement-sensitive (A beta) fibers and from the smaller pain (A delta and C) fibers. Rubbing the painful area stimulates the large movement-sensitive fibers (those that respond to tactile stimulation of the skin and movement of the muscles and joints but not to painful sensation). This inhibits the cells in the spinal cord that transmit the pain message from the small C fibers, and so the message in the cord is decreased before it reaches the brain.

Children learn very quickly that if you gently rub a sore leg, it feels better more rapidly than if you don't rub it. By rubbing the injured site, the child activates a pain "gating" mechanism.

Another way to activate large fibers is to use a TENS unit (see Chapter 6). This technique, developed by Drs. Melzack and Wall, consists of a battery-powered beeper-sized unit with electrodes that are placed on the skin near or within the painful site. The unit blocks the pain signal before it reaches the brain. Pain relief can sometimes continue for several hours after the unit has been turned off.

Gating in the brain

Biofeedback clearly illustrates how the brain can "gate" physiological functions previously considered outside voluntary control, such as heart rate and body temperature. A body signal, such as heart rate, muscle tension, or temperature, is electrically monitored and fed back to that person so that the signal can be altered in a beneficial way. Children have been successfully trained to use biofeedback techniques to alter their biological functions, such as decreasing the tension in the forehead (frontalis) muscle to relieve tension headaches, increasing fingertip temperature to help manage a migraine headache, and increasing rectal sphincter control for bowel problems. (see Chapter 6, p.139) Biofeedback conveys in a measurable way to children and adults the reality of brain-body interaction.

The role of emotions in gating pain

It is now thought that mood is generated in the limbic system, deep in the center of the brain. Mood and emotions interact with many other systems in the human body, and alterations in mood can regulate—increase or decrease—the experience of pain. Here, three children of the same age have a similar leg injury, but their different moods and circumstances change their pain experience.

Child number 1 with a sore leg is excitable and stimulated by the adult attention and direction she is getting. Her stimulation increases the amount of activity going through her nervous system, potentially leading to a greater response to the pain. Since this child's attention is directed to a pop-up book that she finds interesting, she is able to distract herself from her sore leg for a few minutes. Her shift of attention temporarily closes the gate on the full processing of the pain signal in her brain, and she is not very bothered by the pain during that time. Without this alternate focus, the child would feel the pain more intensely. We sometimes hear of this response during sports events: only when the game is finished does an athlete feel the pain of the injury that has occurred earlier in the game. The selected and directed use of attention is the principle behind cognitive-behavioral techniques that include imagery and distraction.

Child number 2 is excitable but also anxious. He is not absorbed in anything other than the pain. His excitability, which is seen in his quick reactions, combines with his anxiety, leading to a greater responsiveness to the pain signals. This child may become more intensely focused on the pain, watching every aspect of his pain, the people involved, and the physical sensations that he is experiencing. His anxiety releases adrenaline and other substances, all of which heighten the child's sensitivity to the pain signals and his reactions and expression of pain. The pain gates in his brain are wide open, allowing all of the pain information to flood into his cortex, and in all likelihood, he feels more pain than child number 1.

Child number 3, in contrast to both previous children, has had leg pain for several months, which has interfered with sports and other loved activities. This child feels disappointed, frustrated, and despairing that her leg will never be the same again. When a person is depressed, the pain gates in the brain tend to stay more widely open, allowing pain to be perceived more fully. The pain leads to greater fatigue, feelings of hopelessness, and depression. We now know that neurotransmitter substances, such as serotonin, become depleted with depression, and this depletion in turn increases the experience of pain. Since this child's pain remains undertreated or is poorly managed, she may also be in a depression-pain cycle, where the persistent pain tires her and increases her feelings of hopelessness, maintaining her brain's responsiveness to the pain signal in her leg.

Antidepressant medication in low or normal doses is therefore very helpful in treating persistent pain that may have caused irritability, anxiety, and interrupted sleep and eating patterns—even if the child or adult is not overtly depressed. Such medication can relieve both pain and its associated problems. Antidepressants can also alter the transmission of painful impulses caused by direct damage to nerves (neuropathic pain), which occurs with spinal cord injuries, and the loss of neuro-muscular function resulting from cancer chemotherapy treatments.

ENDOGENOUS OPIOIDS

What are the specific pain control systems in our brain? In the 1970s, electrical brain stimulation began to be used in humans as an experimental treatment for chronic pain. Electrically stimulating the area behind the thalamus called the periaqueductal gray (PAG), researchers were able to activate a powerful pain control system, blocking pain messages from the spinal cord to the cortex. Today, however, these neurosurgical techniques are not regarded as a panacea for problematic pain, for not only can the pain return but the surgery itself can worsen the pain.

Through the studies, though, it became evident that the electrical stimulation of the PAG activated the same brain mechanisms as morphine, an opioid analgesic medication that is used to treat severe pain, such as pain after surgery. How do morphine and other opioids provide such powerful pain control? The short answer is that they produce pain relief by mimicking the action of the brain's own opioid system (our endogenous opioids).

In the last two decades scientists have discovered that our bodies are capable of producing our own opioids (endorphins) and that we have receptors for these opioids throughout our peripheral and central nervous systems. Dr. Christoph Stein, an anesthesiologist at Johns Hopkins University, has demonstrated that many cells of the immune system also synthesize endorphins. In the presence of inflammation, for example, the immune system can mobilize cells that travel to the site of injury, releasing endorphins, which reduce the transmission of pain.

We now know that when morphine is injected into the bloodstream it travels to the brain, binding with opioid receptors in the PAG and turning on the same pain control system that was activated by electrical brain stimulation. Since the brain and other organs, including the stomach and bowel, have opioid receptors, pain control isn't the only effect that is produced by opioids such as morphine. Severe adverse effects, including lowered blood pressure, constipation, and depression of the respiratory, cardiovascular, and gastrointestinal systems also occur and need to be taken into account when morphine is used (see pages 185–86).

HYPNOSIS

Hypnosis also changes the experience of pain. Achieved through narrowed attention and focused concentration, hypnosis is an altered state of consciousness. During a hypnotic trance, the subject focuses on shrinking, altering, or distancing himself or herself from the pain and, through this process, changes the perception of pain. Children can become skilled at using hypnosis for many different injuries, illnesses, and treatments: burns, cancer, chronic headaches, asthma, wart removal, enuresis, tics, and eczema management. Physiologically, hypnosis, which reduces pain and, in a few instances, entirely blocks pain, seems to work quite differently from medication that acts at sites in the spinal cord and brain. Hypnotic pain control is a fascinating example of how our pain systems do not faithfully transmit the pain signal from the source of injury to the brain.

In experiments on how hypnosis alters pain, Dr. Ernest Hilgard, a psychologist at Stanford University, found that under hypnotic suggestion his adult patients reported out loud that a normally painful sensation to the arm was not painful. Dr. Hilgard then asked the patients, who were still in hypnotic trance, whether a part of their consciousness had noted any pain. Their subconscious, or a part of their brain not involved in the hypnotic process, which Hilgard called the "hidden observer," responded by automatic unconscious writing that severe pain was indeed being experienced. The pain signal got through to the brain, but because of the hypnotic trance it was not deemed "pain" or perceived as "painful."

Children who have been trained to use hypnosis report the same experience. Eight-year-old Seanna, who was in a light hypnotic trance while an IV catheter was being placed into a vein in her hand, remarked: "I know the pain is there, but somehow it doesn't bother me anymore!" Clearly her brain altered the experience of the pain, which, before hypnosis, had greatly hurt and upset her.

ANALGESIC MEDICATIONS

Pain, particularly severe pain, is best controlled and managed by analgesic medication. The medications that are available for use in homes and in hospital are covered in detail in chapter 7. Following is a brief examination of how these commonly used analgesics work in the body.

Acetaminophen, one of the most popular analgesics for use in homes, is used to lower temperature and to provide pain relief. Although it is widely available and generally safely used, scientists still do not know exactly how it achieves both peripheral and central pain relief.

Aspirin, known for its anti-inflammatory properties, can relieve pain in inflamed tissue by halting the synthesis of prostaglandins, inflammatory substances. Its action is thus primarily at the peripheral nerve sites, although recent studies suggest that aspirin may have broader action. Aspirin is one of many non-steroidal anti-inflammatory drugs (NSAIDs), which work mostly at the site of the pain by counteracting the chemicals that promote pain transmission.

Corticosteroids, although not primarily analgesics, can also be used to control pain, particularly cancer pain. Potent anti-inflammatory agents, they work by blocking chemical reactions earlier in the pathway for synthesis of prostaglandins. If taken over a long time, they have serious side effects, such as interfering with bone growth, elevating blood pressure, and interfering with blood glucose control.

Opioids, such as morphine, a synthetic compound derived from the poppy plant, which produces opium, work mainly in the brain and spinal cord in two ways: (1) they decrease the pain message sent to the brain by inhibiting the nerve cells in the spinal cord that receive C nerve fiber messages, and (2) they alter the manner in which the brain perceives the pain stimulus. By binding to the brain's opioid receptors, opioids activate the powerful descending inhibitory control systems that shut down the transmission of pain messages in the spinal cord. These receptors are also used by the body through its own endorphins and enkephalins, which are very short-acting natural pain relievers.

Opioids are effective for severe acute pain, post-surgery pain, pain during medical procedures, and pain related to cancer, AIDS, and sickle cell disease. They create a feeling of distance from the pain, and so there is less awareness of the pain. Opioids can provide significant pain relief, but because opioid receptors occur in many organs of the body and brain, they do produce some side effects, such as lowered blood pressure (usually associated with rapid administration), constipation, and slowing of the respiratory and gastrointestinal systems.

Spinal injections of morphine (epidurals) can block pain for up to 24 hours, whereas the same dose given through the bloodstream will control pain for only three or four hours. As a result, spinal injections of morphine are now commonly used in children's hospitals throughout North America. Although this method produces very good pain relief, especially for certain surgical procedures, it is not a panacea. The opioids infiltrated into the fluid surrounding the spinal cord can travel up to the brain, producing unpleasant side effects, such as nausea, vomiting, itching, and urinary retention. Spinal opioids can, however, also be mixed with local anesthetics, adding to their pain coverage and allowing them to be more effective in combating the pain from certain surgical procedures, injuries, or invasive diseases.

In conclusion, pain is much more than a physiological stimulus; it is an integrated body-brain message, drawing on previous experiences, current mood, beliefs and attitudes, as well as the context and current meaning of the pain. Exactly how pain signals travel from the thalamus into the cerebral cortex and where the final decision is made to declare something "painful" remain a scientist's challenge for the next century.

PART II

How to Relieve Pain

CHAPTER 5

Assessing and Measuring Pain

ATTEMPTING TO ASSESS AND MEASURE another person's pain is like trying to speak a foreign language that you don't understand. When you are in pain you know what is happening, even if it defies accurate expression. When someone else is in pain you can only observe, sympathize, and rely on guesses. To throw a bridge across this chasm, researchers and clinicians in the area of pain have designed a number of instruments to attempt to measure adults' and children's pain. The task is a difficult one: these tools cannot tell the whole story of a child's pain. They can, however, provide a true measure of some aspect of the pain, if only its intensity. A few of these measures are effective for use at home or in hospital with children and adolescents.

Assessing Pain

INFANTS

How infants understand their pain

Infants in the first few months of life do not experience themselves as separate from their mothers or primary caregivers. They assume that when they are in pain their caretaker will immediately know that. They are totally dependent on their caregivers, and they are, therefore, exceptionally vulnerable.

Beginning in the womb and after birth, infants understand and experience the world through their bodies. Their distress is soothed by being held, cuddled, rocked, or comforted with familiar touch and smells; their hunger is sated by the familiar taste of milk. Through the first months of life, infants develop an emerging sense of self and separation from the primary caregiver through a variety of experiences with their bodies (touch, sight, sound, smell, and taste) and a variety of activities.

By six months of age, babies have learned a great deal through their bodies. We know that six-month-old babies who have previously experienced needles as part of their medical treatment will become fearful and actively avoid the anticipated pain. The cry of an infant who sees a person in a white coat with a needle may be an urgent request for help. Over the first year of life, new faces and strange experiences, particularly those of pain, can be deeply disturbing, disrupting infants' willingness to sleep and to eat, and their ability to feel safe and to separate from their parents.

What to look for with infants in pain

With infants, there is no single behavior that is an absolute sign of pain. The best way of judging whether your baby is in pain is to compare what you recognize as your baby's normal behavior with changes in eating, sleeping, moving, and crying. Infants tend to cry if they are in pain and may attempt to pull a sore limb away or to protect a painful area. The facial expression of an infant in pain may look like a grimace, with open mouth and taut cupped tongue. If an infant is in severe pain, however, after first crying, he may become very still, not moving or kicking, and may even stop crying, as if protecting the painful area and conserving energy. Assessment of pain in an infant requires skill. If your infant does not look normal or behave normally, or if there is a fever, consult a physician immediately. Convey to your child's physician the day-to-day changes in behavior that you have noted.

TODDLERS
How toddlers understand pain

Toddlers develop an understanding of their world through their bodies' movements and their senses. From 13 months to approximately 24 months of age, it is very common for children to regard their skin as defining their being. Little wonder that they should be terrified if their skin is punctured or scratched. If the blood all came flowing out—that would be the end! At this age toddlers can't necessarily articulate this fear, but pediatricians have noted toddlers' pre-occupation with wounds and how startled and fearful they are on seeing their blood. Their experiences are still strongly sensory based: *seeing is believing.*

What to look for with toddlers in pain

The first and most helpful step is to ask your toddler directly if she is in pain, or if a suspected part of her body is hurting. Even at one year of age, a toddler can tell you if a part of her body is in pain. Toddlers may not be able to identify their feelings, but if you supply the needed words, young children can correctly identify where and how much they are hurting. Attentiveness and a little patience greatly help in determining this. As with infants, changes in the toddler's normal pattern of moving, behaving, eating, and sleeping may indicate that she is ill or in pain. Unusual behaviors, such as whining or listlessness, may indicate discomfort. Repeatedly tugging at her ear may indicate an ear infection; not putting much weight on a limb or not using an arm could indicate pain or injury.

PRESCHOOLERS
How preschoolers understand pain

Preschool children, aged three to five, regard pain as "something that hurts." As with younger children, the hurting can be overwhelmingly distressing, but, in contrast, preschoolers have many simple words they can use to describe their experience. Children aged three to five understand that there is more to our bodies than outer skin and that beneath their skin there are bones, which the child can easily feel through the skin. They accept the existence of a heart, brain, and other organs commonly talked about; preschool children's understanding of cause and effect and of how their bodies work, however, is very different from an adult's. For example, for the preschooler, the surface—that is, the skin—is still more important than the interior of the body.

Moreover, for children this age, the boundaries between fantasy and reality are blurred. A four-year-old boy runs around the house in an imaginary world, answering to no other name than Robin Hood. A minor hurt in reality becomes a huge fear (remember Hailey, who caught her finger in the three-ringed binder and cried inconsolably for 25 minutes until a Band-aid was found?). Preschoolers will find any reason to "explain" why there is still pain, jumbling up cause and effect. Even if it has been explained once, preschool children don't always understand why they are experiencing pain, what has caused their pain, and how long it will last. The here and now is everything. They have not yet developed an adult's concept of time. Today is still the center of the world, and a week's time is often very difficult to understand ("How many sleeps is it?").

Preschool children need concrete and graphic explanations, repeated and adjusted over time if their pain continues. They need physical proof that pain will come to an end; "two minutes" may not have much meaning to a three-year-old, but holding a Band-aid while having blood drawn means it will soon end, particularly if the child has had some previous experience. Although children as young as three can reliably use some of the pain assessment tools, they still experience themselves as the center of the world, and they may create magic explanations for why the pain is continuing—"maybe because I was naughty." Using drawings, playdough, and other creative tools can be very helpful in determining how preschool children understand and deal with their pain.

What to look for with preschoolers in pain

When a preschooler has the words to describe his experiences, question the child about the nature of his pain. You should also observe his movements and behavior and note any changes in his regular eating and sleeping patterns. Encourage the young child to express what he is experiencing and attempt to understand how he is interpreting the pain signals. Remember that children of this age often think magically (it is the age of imaginary friends and monsters that live under the bed). Assure the child that he did not get the pain because he did something wrong or is being punished but that infections, accidents, and pain occur and that he can help himself feel better by following the pain treatment program. A vital part of this stage of development is gaining increased mastery and understanding of events. This development is reflected in the fact that preschool children can actively use coping skills that demonstrate self-control and the ability to modify their pain.

SCHOOL-AGED CHILDREN
How school-aged children understand pain

In their early school years, from 6 to 12 years of age, children tend to regard pain in a general fashion. They draw on internal cues to determine whether they are sick, but they are often still naive about external causes, such as infections. Children may still think that pain is a consequence of their bad behavior or a form of punishment. School-aged children, however, are more capable of logic than preschoolers, even though their understanding of the link between cause and effect is still fairly concrete. With the use of books, drawings, and charts, school-aged children can begin to conceptualize pain occurring in their bodies and learn about the nervous system and how body and brain send and receive pain signals. Children at school are often familiar with computers, which can provide a good analogy for how the brain functions, remembering and making sense of the current and previous painful experiences. When the adults in school-aged children's lives take the time to discuss and explain matters and to clear up misconceptions, these children are much better able to understand and manage their pain.

What to look for with school-aged children in pain

With their greater language skills and understanding of different situations, school-aged children are usually more consistent in their expressions of pain than younger children. Thus, it is much easier to identify when a child is in pain. Once again, changes in eating, activity level, and ways of moving and behaving can be signs of the presence of pain. Asking the child directly and talking over what you have observed and what your child is experiencing will provide crucial information. Note that at this age boys may have become more stoic or inexpressive of their pain than girls and therefore may require more attention.

TEENAGERS

How teenagers understand pain

By the age of 12 or 13, adolescents are capable of thinking abstractly: they can reflect on their own thoughts in more flexible and systematic ways. Teens often show insight into the psychological factors or consequences of their pain. These are the years of becoming more of an individual, not only in clothing and looks, but also in beliefs and attitudes, as well as in personal experiences of pain. By 11 to 14 years and onward, teenagers have acquired some knowledge of how pain works and often realize the value of pain as a protective and warning signal. But they may also have learned unhelpful responses to pain, such as ignoring the pain signals. Under the stress of pain, teenagers, like all children, can regress to younger ways of behaving.

What to look for with teens in pain

The indicators of pain are very similar to those of school-aged children, who are able to identify the site, type, onset, and intensity of pain. When in the presence of their friends, however, teenagers may adopt different behaviors and may talk very differently about their pain. If observed by friends, teenagers tend to minimize or deny their pain. To gather a true picture of a teenager's pain, it is crucial to have a private discussion so that peer pressures can not come into play and distort the teen's reporting.

Measuring Pain

We face a dilemma when we attempt to measure a person's pain, in that the forms of measurement we use are imperfect. One form—what the person in pain reports—is subjective, and the other form—what the person looking on observes—is considered objective. Although the subjective report is the most important, since the pain is that person's experience, each measure has its strengths and weaknesses. The subjective measurement has the authenticity of an eyewitness report, but it is colored by, for example, culture, family history, and previous pain experiences (see *figure 4.4*). The observer's report purports to be objective—but is there a pure objective stance devoid of that person's emotions, attitudes, and previous experience? Moreover, the subjective measure and the objective measure may not fit—in fact, sometimes they may provide two different pictures. As an example, you notice a child limping and not using his leg properly, as if his leg may be hurting. When asked about this, the child denies having any leg pain. Clearly, something doesn't fit. More information, observation, and gentle questioning are needed.

A third form of measuring pain is the direct measurement of the body's functions, using indices such as the heart beat, degree of sweating, or respiration rate. Unfortunately, these indices do not tell us in a consistent and dependable way about the presence, absence, or intensity of pain. In short, there is no reliable direct measure, or combination of measures of pain. For example, acute pain may increase respiration rate, heart rate, sweating, and hormonal changes. When pain persists over time, however, as in a chronic pain condition, the pain may be severe, but these physiological responses do not necessarily occur. Once again we are faced with the complexity of pain: pain is not one reaction or emotional response or behavior; rather, it is a multifactored, complex experience of mind and body to which our systems adapt and adjust.

Measuring pain in young, pre-verbal children adds another level of challenge to the problem. Adults in pain usually speak up for themselves and describe in detail the nature of their pain. Children, who have limited life experiences, feel overwhelmed and scared and do not have the language or interpersonal skills to speak for themselves or to insist on being heard. With very young children and infants, who are not yet able to use language to convey where and how much they are in pain, measuring their pain becomes a major hurdle, requiring experience and considerable knowledge of infant behavior. Toward the end of the first year of life, as children begin to communicate with words, their own report of pain, for many reasons, becomes the first and most important way of knowing that they are in pain. Thus, self-report measures become a particularly important form of measuring pain.

REASONS FOR USING SOME FORM OF MEASUREMENT

There are a number of sound reasons to attempt to measure or quantify a child's pain. First, such an attempt builds a communication bridge, conveying useful details. For example, a child who has frequent headache pain may usually say the pain is five on a scale of ten. When there are some changes, instead of saying, "It is worse" or "It is a little better," this child is able to say, "It's now a six out of ten." Health care staff or parents can then enquire when it started to move up or down the scale and find out more about the many factors that aggravate or ease the pain.

Second, by using an established tool, child, parent, and staff can determine the success of the pain intervention. For example, half an hour after using a hypnosis tape combined with cold cloth on her head, the child can report whether the pain has changed. If the change is in the right direction, down, and the child feels it is helping, the method can be continued. If, however, the pain remains the same, decreases insignificantly, or increases, then it is clear that another method should be considered.

Third, when children experience recurring or persistent pain, the consistent use of measures becomes a more finely tuned language by which the child can quickly and reliably learn to convey changes in pain over time. Using this language bridge provides security to the child in pain; he no longer feels so isolated when pain absorbs his energy and attention, for his caregivers will know the difference between his rating of a three and a six out of ten. With these increased communication skills, caregivers tend to respond more promptly and, where needed, to provide pain medication.

Measuring a child's pain also involves knowing the number of times the pain occurred (frequency), the length of time it lasted (duration), and how strong it was (intensity). All three are very helpful in determining the effectiveness of the method selected to reduce the child's pain. Noting the different levels of pain can also assist in determining the various triggers of the pain. Remember that a child's (or adult's) report of pain is a private and personal rating that is unique to that person. Comparing one child's ratings to another's has no validity and should not be done. We can only make meaningful comparisons between the same child's ratings on different occasions.

A CAUTION

Children are sensitive to their environment, and this sensitivity affects how they report their pain. Some children, wanting to please the person who is asking them questions, may say what they think the person wants to hear. Others may be fearful of certain consequences—for example, separation from their parents—and thus will under-report their pain. Under-reporting of pain frequently occurs in new and uncertain situations, like hospitals. Parents are usually very good at sensing what is really happening and can encourage the child to say what he or she is really experiencing.

The following section describes the various tools to use with children of different ages to obtain their self-report of pain.

TOOLS FOR A CHILD'S OWN REPORT OF PAIN

These tools are either quantitative (using numbers) or qualitative (conveying the details, colors, shapes, and context of the pain experience). The number scales are easy to use and are a good place to start in determining what is happening in the child's pain. Be aware, however, that these are not very sensitive measures and will not tell you a great deal about the child's full personal experience. The qualitative measures, such as drawings and diaries, are more complex, rich, and variable, and so comparisons over time are trickier, since they are more open to subjective interpretations. Nevertheless, they provide an excellent avenue for appreciating and discussing the pain experience with a child.

Try out some of the following tools ahead of time to ascertain which ones your child finds most interesting. You should also experiment to find out which tools are the most useful to you when your child is in pain.

Poker Chips (figure 5.1)

Age: 4 to 8 years

Developed by: Dr. Nancy Hester, nursing professor in Colorado

Use four red poker chips, if you have them, or any red pieces of the same sizes. One means a tiny bit of pain; two, a little more pain; three, still more pain; and four, the most pain of all. Ask your child how many "pieces of hurt" she has. This is a simple, concrete tool that is very useful

Figure 5.1

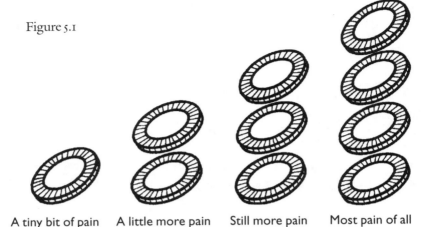

A tiny bit of pain   A little more pain   Still more pain   Most pain of all

with young children in pain. It is easy for children to understand and to use to arrive at a decision.

Children's Anxiety and Pain Scale (CAPS) (figure 5.2)

Age: 4 to 10 years
Developed by: Dr. Leora Kuttner and Dr. Tony Le Page, pediatric psychologists in Vancouver, Canada

Face scales, either as cartoons or more detailed faces, are popular and useful, since facial expressions convey a lot of information and are quick and easy for children to understand. The faces are shown to the child, and the child is asked to choose which face shows how much pain he is having. The Children's Anxiety and Pain Scale (CAPS) consists of two face scales, one to determine anxiety, the other to determine the level of pain. Since anxiety can confound the measuring of pain, it is best to start with the anxiety scale. To orient the child to the scale, say to the child that these faces show how scared the child is when he is in pain, pointing to each face as you explain what it shows. The first face shows that this child is not scared, the second face shows that this child is a tiny bit scared, the third face shows that this child is a little more scared, the fourth shows that the child is quite a lot scared, and the fifth face shows that the child is very, very scared. Ask the child to point to the face that shows how scared he feels.

Turning to the pain scale, orient the child by saying that these faces show how much pain a child is having. Go through the faces as before; once again, the first indicates that the child is in no pain; the second,

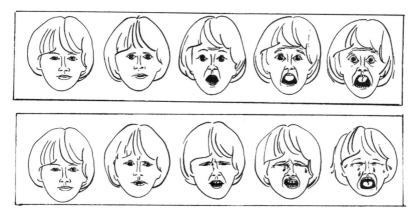

Figure 5.2 *Childrens's Anxiety and Pain Scale (CAPS)*

that the child is feeling a little pain; the third, that the child is experiencing a little more pain; the fourth, that the child feels quite a lot of pain; and the last, that the child feels a great deal of pain. Ask the child to point to the face that shows the amount of pain he is experiencing.

Pain Thermometer (figure 5.3)

Age: 6 and older

We don't know who developed this widely used measure—one of the most useful for all ages. Once it is learned, it can become an easy shorthand form of communication. Children are used to the idea of a thermometer, and having one that measures pain is an easy concept to grasp. Once again, orient the child to the thermometer, indicating that the 0 at the bottom shows that there is no pain. Going up the scale, 1 is a little pain, 3 is quite a bit of pain, 5 is even more, 7 is quite a lot of pain, 9 is a great deal of pain, and 10 is the worst pain you have ever had or could ever imagine having. Ask the child, "Where are *you* on this scale right now?" or "How much pain are you in?"

A child or teen can then easily carry the idea of the vertical pain thermometer in her head. After a time you may not need to draw it for the child, but can simply say, "On the pain thermometer, how much pain do you have now?" Then keep a record of the score, time, and date. Remember that the child's self-ratings should only be compared with her own previous ratings. In figure 5.3, the pain thermometer has been labeled "before" and "after" to show on the same thermometer the measure before providing a method of pain relief, and the measure after the

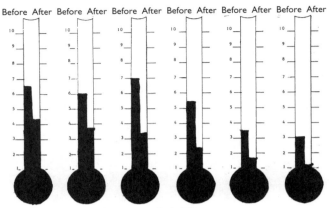

Figure 5.3 *Pain Thermometer*

method was used. A before-and-after measure helps gauge the effectiveness of the method. Some hospitals find these scores so useful that they routinely record the child's self-reported pain score out of ten on the child's bed chart, together with pulse, heart rate, and other vital signs.

Pain Diary (figure 5.4)

Age: 6 and older

Pain diaries can be designed for each child's particular circumstance. The diary should include regular recordings of the date and time the pain occurred, the pain intensity rating (how bad it was), what happened before the pain started, how the pain was treated, and how suc-

Figure 5.4

Date				
Time				
Pain level Scale: 1–10				
Activity when pain began				
What helped relieve it				
How long it took to get comfortable				
Pain level now				

Figure 5.5

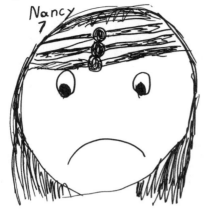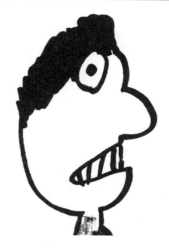

Recurrent migraine-tension headaches drawn by a seven-year-old girl

Tension headache drawn by a nine-year-old boy

cessful the treatment was. Children in the first few years of school (six to eight years old) may need some help completing the diary. As a record, the pain diary can reveal patterns during the day, week, and month, as well as what other events may contribute to the pain. The diary is an especially helpful tool if the child's pain is puzzling or if it is a recurring pain that needs to be better understood and better managed.

Drawings (figure 5.5)
All ages

A child's or teen's own drawing of pain provides one of the best and most evocative means of understanding what he is going through when in pain. It also concisely conveys a great deal of information about the qualities of the pain experience. The colors, forms, and style that the child uses in the drawing, as well as the intensity of the drawing, provide important information. Above all, the drawing can be the starting point for a discussion with the child to better understand his pain.

Eland Body Tool (figure 5.6)
Age: 5 years and older
Developed by: Dr. Jo Eland, nursing professor, Iowa

Children relate very easily to the children's figures in these diagrams, especially since they have some clothes on. Children, it seems, are more prepared to indicate where their pain is occurring if the figure has

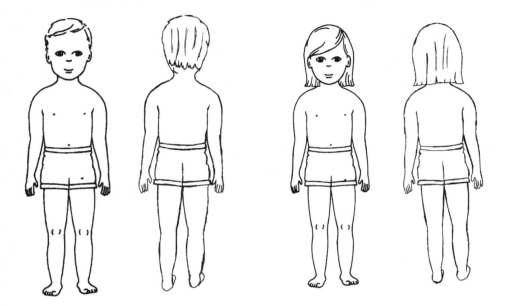

Figure 5.6 *The Eland Body Tool*

clothes on than if it does not. Notice that there is a back to the figures, which is helpful in gaining a full picture of the extent of the child's pain. A fuller, more complex view of the child's pain can be achieved if you ask the child to select a color that shows the most pain, another color for a medium amount of pain, and a third color for the least pain. Then ask the child to color the body with each of the three colors, depicting where the worst pain, medium pain, and least pain are occurring. Once again, if this tool is used repeatedly over time, it can show a picture of the changes that occur.

Conclusion

The most common question that children in pain are asked is, "How is your pain today?" Such a vague question is not of great benefit to either the child or the clinician. In fact, often in the hospital this broad question becomes a health professional's social pleasantry on entering the child's room. It would be more helpful if, after a genuine hello, the child were questioned as follows: "Would you tell me about your pain? Can you measure your pain today on your scale or with your chips so that I can know how much pain you still have?" "Using those body maps again, show me where your pain is now, and using your colors show me how your pain feels."

The child's responses may provide useful information in tracking and treating the pain; we know that these responses are far from simple, however. The report of pain is influenced by many factors, including the child's mood, desire to please, fatigue or state of the disease, cultural and family norms, and perception of the current situation. In other words, the condition causing the pain is but one of the contributors to the experience of pain, as shown in figure 4.3. Nevertheless, the child's own report of the pain experience is the most important place to start in the evaluation of this pain over time.

Not all children at home need to have their pain measured, but some assessment is helpful if you are going to provide a method of pain relief. Perhaps the pain thermometer and the pain diary are most convenient for children at home with recurring or persistent pain, for these tools reveal the intensity and the pattern of the pain, both of which are central concerns when you are looking for methods to relieve pain.

CHAPTER 6

Methods to Help Relieve Pain

*It's not that we don't know what to do when a child is in pain. We do,
but we don't always do it.*

— DR. DON TYLER, PAIN DIRECTOR AND
ANESTHESIOLOGIST, SEATTLE CHILDREN'S HOSPITAL

THIS CHAPTER DESCRIBES TECHNIQUES that will help a child
who is in pain and distressed. Most of the techniques draw on the everyday experiences of children, teenagers, and parents. You do not have to
be a nurse or a doctor to apply most of these techniques. Children naturally think in images, breathe in different rhythms at different times of
the day, adore playing with bubbles and ice, enjoy sucking popsicles, often request a back rub, love to hear stories, and relax easily with a heating pad or in a warm bath. Most children know the difference between
helpful thoughts and the kind of thinking that aggravates pain. Children also like to have some control over what happens to them and will
willingly divert their attention to something more interesting, if they
trust that it will help them through the pain. When used promptly to relieve pain, distress, and anxiety, these methods, with or without suitable
medication, will become a natural part of your child's strategy for coping with sudden, sharp pain or with achy, persistent pain.

An important note: If you are unsure about the nature of your child's
pain, do not use the methods outlined in this chapter *in place of* having a
physician conduct a thorough medical investigation of your child's
pain. Some causes of pain could be infectious or malignant and there-

fore require and respond well to medical intervention. It is important to have a good clinical evaluation of pain to assess any pain that is unusual, persistent, or difficult to explain. Once you know what you're dealing with, you can use the best therapeutic method, or combination of methods, suitable for the pain.

The pain-relieving methods listed in this chapter are easy to use with your child and can be fine-tuned over time. None of these methods is exclusive, and all work harmoniously with each other. In fact, when combined they reinforce each other, providing a more comprehensive treatment. For example, if a child in severe pain focuses on the image of her pain becoming smaller and deliberately relaxes her body at the same time that pain medication is being delivered, she is likely to achieve more comprehensive relief from pain and suffering than from medication on its own or the sole use of relaxation or imagery. Discuss your therapeutic choices with your physician to ensure that your choice of method is best suited to your child's pain and to share with him or her your approach to your child's pain management.

Table 6.1 Methods of Relieving Pain

Language That Helps Pain to Go	Breathing Methods
Touch	Breathing-Relaxation Methods
Massage	Imagery
Therapeutic Touch	Combining Pain Imagery with Medication
Ice	Hypnosis
Water	Biofeedback
Heat	Music
Ice and Heat	Play and Art
Acupuncture	Control
Acupressure	
TENS	
Carrying, Rapid Rocking, and Sucking a Pacifier	

Table 6.1 lists all the methods discussed in this chapter. A few of the methods are more high-tech than others and initially require a trained professional. For example, the TENS unit, which can be used at home, will initially require the guidance of a physiotherapist, nurse, or physician (help is usually offered when the unit is rented or bought). Acupuncture

is a highly trained science and art form performed by acupuncturists, who are often also trained medical practitioners. Acupressure is usually practiced by massage therapists or physiotherapists. Biofeedback relies on complex, costly machines, knowledge, and skill, and hypnosis should be taught by a health professional, such as a psychologist, doctor, nurse, or social worker trained in pain management and hypnotic methods. The full range of methods is included here to inform you of their use and application in pain management. If you decide that they will be of help, you can find a children's health professional with the specific skill needed.

Guiding Principles for Using Methods of Relieving Pain

Remind your child that the pain will get better. As you start using a new method, keep alive the hope that the pain will get better. When the pain begins to ease, ask exactly how the pain got better and what helped the child the most

Give your child control. Let him choose the methods that work best or the way they should be used or combined (further ways of giving a child control are discussed later on in this chapter).

Be flexible in applying these methods. Since children have different temperaments, preferences, and levels of pain tolerance, what works for one child may not work for another.

If the first experience doesn't work, don't throw everything out. Find out what your child enjoyed, which parts helped, and which parts didn't work. Build on the parts that helped: "Since the relaxing part didn't work, how about sitting up this time when we use the music with that hang-gliding imagery?"

Encourage the child to take over the method and make it her own. Support any tentative steps in that direction. As the child moves from being passive recipient to playing a more active role in shaping and developing treatment, she will tailor it to her needs and her pain. The changes that occur can be dramatic and have a long-range impact on her self-concept and her life.

Use language and ideas that invite hope and courage. Children in pain quickly feel defeated. Thus, you might say: "I suspect you'll find the CT scan much better when you use your thought-stopping," "You *can* make it better. Remember how you felt when you first rode your two-wheel bike, after thinking you would never be able to do it?"

Pay close attention to the child's facial expressions, positions, and movements throughout the experience. Non-verbal cues are as important as verbal ones. If you sense that something is amiss, check with the child: "Is this okay with you?" Or "What do you need now to make it better?" Your watchful support frees the child to enter the experience more fully and to draw the needed relief.

Encourage regular, daily practice of these methods if possible, since it strengthens the effect, benefits, and changes.

Methods of Relieving Pain
LANGUAGE THAT HELPS PAIN TO GO

Language that conveys any degree of support, hope, love, courage, energy, or affection, and that promises at least some release from suffering helps children to let go of their fear and pain. Therapeutic language goes hand in hand with attentive listening. As you actively attend to a child's language and behavior, you teach yourself to respond to his or her messages. As you exchange messages through language and tone with the child in pain, you also convey your own attitudes. In other words: what you say and how you say it reflects what you think, as well as what you believe, what you teach, what you expect, and even at times what is likely to happen. Here are some useful pointers for using language therapeutically with a child in pain.

This section on language was written with Dr. Dan Kohen, director, Behavioral Pediatrics Program and associate professor of pediatrics, Family Practice and Community Health, University of Minnesota. Dr. Kohen and I have a long and successful association, teaching pediatric staff through the Society of Behavioral Pediatrics how to use hypnosis to help children with their problems.

How *you talk is as important as* what *you say* Depending on how urgent a situation may be, how you talk—your manner, tone of voice, and intonation—conveys the degree to which you believe what you are saying. All of the features of the message are conveyed automatically to your child, who knows you so well. Children tell us when we sound silly, serious, funny, angry, or not particularly believable. Sometimes we are surprised when they say, "You sound angry," or "you sound upset," because perhaps we didn't even realize how we were talking, much less precisely what we said. We are lucky if our children tell us these things at these times; often they are not conscious of their response to what we say and how we have said it. We then see the effects of that message in the child's subsequent behavior and responses.

1. *Acknowledge and ask about the pain.* You can help a great deal by simply acknowledging a child's pain: "You are in a lot of pain right now, and we are going to help you," "It is clear that you have had a lot of pain.

Can you tell me about it?" When you ask a child to describe the discomfort very precisely, it helps the child to define the pain and, most important, conveys the idea that he is believed, that you are interested, that you share his concern, that you will not quarrel with it, and that you will continue to help. You can say: "The more I know about your pain, the more I can understand it, and the better I can help. After all, it's your pain and you know it better than I do. Please help me understand it."

At first glance this might seem like focussing too much on the pain, but it helps the child to *compartmentalize* the discomfort, to know not only where it is precisely but everything about it. This "cognitive mastery" is very important for young children, especially, who need to know everything they possibly can about their discomfort. Listening to the child's description allows you to understand more clearly what the child is experiencing, to learn how she is conceptualizing her pain, and it gives you clues about ways you can use words and ideas to help alter her perceptions to her own benefit, to reduce suffering.

2. *Do not underestimate the power of listening.* The other half of the therapeutic impact of language is the therapeutic benefit of listening. As you ask questions, be sure to wait patiently and with positive expectation for the child's answer, which, when given, allows you to explore further and simultaneously to convey some courage or comfort.

3. *Pace this process respectfully.* Even when we are eager to help and to "fix it," remember that obtaining this information should be at a pace and rhythm that works for the child. As you show the child that you can wait, you teach not only sensitivity but also patience by your own example.

4. *Define the child's pain by framing it with hope, not doom.* For a child with multiple lacerations, an example of a statement made to the emergency staff framed with hope might be: "He's an energetic boy. He fell off his skateboard, and it looks as if he'll need some stitches so that he'll heal well." Compare such a response to one laced with guilt, doubts, and doom, "Boy, this is a mess! I wish he never had a skateboard. Lots of stitches? I hope he won't have too many scars!" This response may seem exaggerated, but it is not uncommon. Children listen carefully and watch closely. The first statements they hear may go a long way toward establishing whether they will cope or worry. Therefore, you must select language that invites hope and includes possibilities for the child's improvement.

5. *Reframe the child's distress.* If a child has defined the pain as a catastrophe, you can "reframe" it. For example, a child says, "This pain is killing me!" A positive reframing may begin with an affirmation. For ex-

ample: "It does hurt a lot and your body is clearly saying it is ready for some *powerful* help. Why don't we use your hypnosis tape." This kind of response helps because it offers an alternative without denying the child's experience. When a child is startled and frightened by the sight of her blood, you can reframe the experience by saying, "What beautiful blood you have! It's a wonderful bright strong red. Look! I can tell it's healthy by its color. Your blood is doing a good job of cleaning the wound out. That's excellent. It'll stop very soon." Since using positive language can be very powerful and its effects long-lasting, always make an effort to think about what you say and how you say it.

6. *Replace pain-loaded words with more tolerable words.* What we believe and how we think and talk about pain and suffering are products of how we were brought up and specifically of what experiences we have had personally with discomfort. Did you notice the shift from the word "pain" to the word "discomfort"? Did it change how you reacted? The word "discomfort" holds within it the possibility of comfort. This kind of shift even in single words is an important step in the development of your own conceptual framework of what pain is and is not and, more important, what you believe you can and cannot do in response to it.

Another shift you may wish to employ, especially when talking to a child about previous or recurrent pain, is to refer to an "episode" instead of an "attack" of pain. "Episode" is a neutral word that doesn't suggest hurt. "Attack" is a negative word that implies helplessness and fear and thus has no therapeutic value. You might say to the child: "Let's use 'episode' or 'event' for each time you have had discomfort or when you are 'bothered.' " Most children will accept the invitation to throw out that negative word.

7. *Draw on words that have worked for you.* How you think about pain comes from how you made sense of and navigated uncomfortable pain experiences as a child yourself and how the adults around you responded at those times. As you think of language that eases pain and suffering, you may draw on the phrases you remember adults saying to you that were reassuring or useful. One mother, who had scarlet fever when she was six, a few years before antibiotics were available, recalled how her mother, despite her worry, soothingly said to her, "You want to get better, don't you? You *will* get better; you'll *soon* get better." Remembering the power that her mother's words gave her, this daughter drew on these words again when her nine-year-old Katie was suffering, knowing that they might give her hope and strength.

8. *Note the parts of the body that are not in pain.* If a child is preoccupied with and overfocused on the pain, and not open to coping, you can use language that shifts the child's attention. One day six-year-old Josh was on a picnic with a group of friends. Another boy about his age fell while running and banged his knee. As he sat screaming on the ground holding his knee, Josh was the first one to reach him. As the other adults approached moments later, they heard Josh asking his playmate, "How's your *other* knee?" which had not been injured. In a flash his friend stopped crying, turned his attention to the other knee, and said it was fine, and then they both got up to play.

Shifting attention to where it is not hurting not only can help move a child out of panic or shock but can also be used to delineate the limits of the pain. When the child feels trapped by persistent pain, say: "I know your leg is really sore in traction, with the pin in place after surgery, but is it sore in your hip? No! Good. How about in your back? No! Excellent! And in your ankle? No! I'm very glad to hear this, because it means that the pain is bad from the top of your leg to your calf, but it isn't in your hip, your back, or your ankle. We'll check this again in an hour and see how much it has improved."

Post-surgery situations, such as the one referred to above, require frequent reassessment of the child's pain, for it is imperative to ensure that the child has sufficient pain medication and is not suffering needlessly. Defining the spread of the pain can be one helpful index among many in the assessment of the child's pain.

9. *Use language that implies positive change.* Your own experiences with negativity toward, or helplessness with, pain can spill over into what you come to expect in situations of pain with your children. One day while walking through the general clinic, Dan overheard a little girl about five years old crying and coughing, complaining that her throat "hurt a lot." Her mother, embarrassed by her daughter's commotion, was reprimanding her. Dan asked if the child would tell him about her sore throat. She stopped crying and told him. She was given some acetaminophen for her discomfort and fever and told that her doctor would be in to check her over soon. Before leaving Dan told her, "You'll probably be surprised how fast you start to get better." She calmed down quite readily, for her hurt had been acknowledged and some relief provided. Perhaps just as important, however, was using language that was positive and supportive. Dan's final words of encouragement provided this little girl with hope for change without making false promises

or denying her discomfort. Language like this provides comfort because it diminishes the fear and the uncertainty, which often, if not always, is associated with a child's painful experiences.

10. *Use words of reassurance and encouragement.* You can use words that encourage your child, or provide a little more courage to get through a painful episode. The benefit of having a coach to provide that injection of courage must never be underestimated. "You *can* do it. You're helping your body get more comfortable when you do your breathing-relaxation. I can tell how much better you seem afterwards." Active coaching is tracking and keeping pace with your child, providing the help and encouragement for him to get through the discomfort, without doing it entirely alone.

11. *Where possible, let the child know that what he or she is experiencing is normal and not life-threatening or the result of a terrible disease.* Children have active imaginations and unless correctly informed may imagine the worst: "Your pain feels terrible because your arm is broken and bruised, and the nerves there are hurting and complaining. It helps to know that it is usual for this to happen when a bone breaks. So to ease the nerves, we will immediately give you some medication called codeine. You'll feel much better within a few minutes. Your arm may remain very tender and you'll need to keep it still in this sling, until we set it in a cast. You'll feel like your regular self pretty soon."

12. *Remind the child that the pain will come to an end.* Always truthfully, and whenever possible, provide the child with some idea of how long this pain is likely to last. Tailor this information to the age of the child. For example, for a school-aged child, you could say during a needle insertion, "By the count of ten you'll probably hardly notice it, or it may stop altogether." For a preschool-aged child after surgery, you could say, "After three sleeps you'll be able to get out of bed and the pain won't bother you as much." A general statement that will convey that the pain will come to an end is: "I'm wondering how quickly and easily you'll notice the easing of your discomfort, because children's bodies heal quickly." Pain is rarely a steady, consistent sensation, and in general children's bodies repair and heal much more quickly than do those of adults.

13. *Avoid words that might conjure up fear.* For example, if you say, "Don't be afraid, it won't hurt much," children hear "afraid" and "hurt much." Use words that inspire courage and coping, and sustain the hope that pain will ease.

Which words you use, and when and how you use them, matters a lot. These messages can accompany the many pain-relieving methods described in the rest of this chapter. Using the first method, the various forms of touch, one need not necessarily speak at all, since the quality of touching itself conveys the message of comfort and easing of pain.

TOUCH

Age: Birth and older
Pain: Most forms
Time: As long as desired by the child or parent

Touch by someone who cares can be a comforting, soothing, and healing experience for anyone of any age suffering pain. Touching cuts through the isolation that being in pain brings. A familiar loving sensation is an immediate reminder of love, security, and comfort and can temporarily mask or distract one from the pain sensation. Parents know this intuitively. Unfortunately, the environment of a clinic or the intimidation of hospital protocol sometimes prevents or inhibits parents, brothers, sisters, or grandparents from touching, holding, or stroking the hurting child in the way they wish or the child needs. Sometimes concerns about being brave or grown-up prevent older children from accepting the comfort of touch.

Touching to relieve pain can take many forms, including patting, stroking, and rubbing. The choice depends on the nature of the pain, the child's age, and individual preferences. When someone is in pain, a specific area of the body may be tender, aching, or throbbing. There are usually other areas, however, that are not hurting. If you stroke, pat, tickle, or massage a nonhurting area of your child's body, and the child finds the sensation pleasant, the pleasant sensation will begin to compete with the painful ones for the child's attention. This kind of touching is most effective if it is able to evoke a familiar memory:

Tammy had pain in her throat and was feeling groggy after the anesthetic and her tonsillectomy. As Tammy's mom tickled the sensitive inside of her arm, the familiar sensation immediately informed her that she was not alone: Mom was there. That soothing tickling feeling had a long history, reminding her of lying in comfort in her bed, falling asleep into dreams, with her mom at her side, tickling her arm.

By asking parents what touch the child likes, pediatric personnel can make their therapy more effective. Even when a child is in severe pain, that touch will carry associations of support, relief, and comfort. Children have often said that holding a familiar loving hand during the pain was a lifeline.

Patting can be very soothing for infants, toddlers, and fearful young children. Different children prefer different types of patting, depending on their previous experience. A baby whose parents routinely comfort him by patting his back in a particular way will know that distinctive style and will quickly respond. A stranger patting him with hesitancy or too much vigor may be less successful at helping him. Patting at a rate of about twice a second has been recommended as a natural cadence that stimulates the large movement fibers and inhibits the small pain fibers, providing some relief.

For older children in pain, patting may make them feel infantilized; be guided by your knowledge of the child. Some children who feel vulnerable may find patting a welcome physical distraction from acute or pressing pain. If older children regress to a younger age because of their pain and distress, patting can be soothing and settling, providing an alternative sensation on which to focus. Soothing patting becomes a reminder that the pain isn't completely overwhelming and that the pain has not isolated the child from your caring. It is also a reminder that other parts of her body can feel good.

Stroking can be a favorite; many children love to have their faces stroked or their hair played with, brushed, or repetitively stroked. Stroking in continuous rhythmic motion is more acceptable for older children who have persistent pain. It becomes a distraction from the insistent and unwelcome presence of gnawing and draining pain. Gently stroking a child's face, arms, or back is an immediate reminder that you are there and that you care. Older children often guide their parents: "Dad, stroke me here. No, higher!" Children focus on and become increasingly absorbed by the pleasant sensation of being stroked.

Rubbing can provide physiological benefits (discussed in chapter 4). Rubbing a mild injury stimulates the large muscle and nerve fibers, which in turn inhibit the smaller pain fibers at the spinal cord. A young child could be taught that when he falls, one of the ways to help the pain go away is to rub the sore area in the way that feels best. Children learn very quickly what works. You may be surprised to notice on the next fall a toddler or preschool-aged child rubbing the injured area to ease the pain. Rubbing and simultaneously blowing out (discussed later in this chapter) make a good combination for reducing pain and distress.

MASSAGE

Age: Birth to adult
Pain: Achy muscles, spasms, "growing pains"
Time: As long as needed

Massage helps to relax muscles and to ease spasms and aches. Warm a little lotion or oil in your hands and rub with light, easy, circular sweeps over the sore and painful areas. Teenagers may want firmer pressure. Physiotherapists and massage therapists recommend the use of the fleshy palm of your hand rather than your fingers for better contact with the child's body. Your hand should not leave the child's body until the massage ends so that the child always knows where you are and the contact remains unbroken. As you finish a sweep, allow your fingers to trail gently back up so that your fingertips don't leave the child's skin. Allow your hand to flow around bony points. If you are massaging a child's back, a preferred movement is up the muscle along the spine and then to the sides of the body. Encourage your child to guide you by asking questions, such as "Should I press a little harder here?" or "Do you like it more when I use my fingertips like this, or my palms, like this?" It is best to start off gently until the muscles relax; then increase the intensity to soften the muscles further. Be guided by your child at all times.

Sometimes a warm hand lightly resting on an achy stomach can help the muscles relax and soften. Gentle massage in this location can also be helpful. You can lightly stroke the stomach in concentric circles, going from small to large, or vice versa, from large circles to small ones. Deeper massage of the stomach is seldom helpful and can induce pain.

Seven-year-old Christopher had severe stomach pains. He would have spasms and double over crying. Most of the time he walked around with his arms over his stomach area, protecting it. Over a two-month period he had been thoroughly investigated by his family doctor and a pediatric gastrointestinal specialist, who could find no underlying disease or infection. Yet Christopher's pain continued, as did his reluctance to eat anything solid, apart from oatmeal cereal. A number of methods were used to help Christopher ease his stomach pain, including drawing, play-therapy, imagery-relaxation, gradually extending his range of foods, and massage. Tolerating the massage became proof for Christopher that his tummy was getting better. He had been so scared that anything might start the pain up again that he had not been able to tolerate anyone touching his tummy, let alone massaging it. Gradually, over three weeks of using the different pain-reduction methods, and slowly increasing his foods to include cooked vegetables, fish, and multivitamins and mineral supplements, Christopher began to trust that he did not need to fear the pain. He learned that there were things that his dad and mom and he could do that would help the pain subside. He became stronger and more playful, and his parents reported that he smiled more often. With the reduction in his stomach pain, his massages became transformed into an animal recognition game: his Mom drew patterns of different animals on his tummy, which he would name or guess!

When a child is having mild bowel pain, tenderness, constipation, or gassy pains, use oil with light or slightly deeper small circular motions from the right of the bowel across the belly button to the left and follow the anatomical structure of the bowel in an upside-down U shape. There are often particular sites along the bowel that are more tender than others: if your child finds it agreeable, gently massage the irritable or tender sites a little longer. Older children often prefer massaging themselves, since it enables them to do what feels best.

Although not its primary benefit, massage can also be used to create a competing sensation in a pain-free area that will comfort and distract the child from the pain. While waiting for wounds to heal after surgery, you can massage head, feet, toes (if the child is not too ticklish), or any other area unaffected by pain. For children and teenagers who are very ill and don't have the energy or inclination to talk, massage is a wonderful method of staying connected and providing comfort. Here is how I used it with Jessica.

When Jessica, a spunky teenager, was struggling to recover from a bone-marrow transplant to treat her cancer, her entire body ached from the effects of the treatment. She had developed a physical complication secondary to the transplant: her skin was sloughing off. It hurt to move. Her mouth was filled with ulcers as a result of her weakened immune system. It hurt to talk. Even her eyes were sore. But her feet were okay. She wanted company but no conversation. She softly nodded when I suggested a foot massage. For about ten minutes I gently rubbed and kneaded her feet, massaging her heels and around her ankles, down over the front of her foot to her toes, and gently between each toe. After her release from isolation, she said that foot massage had helped her to concentrate on one good feeling in her body, while the rest of her felt so weak and sore. She thereafter regularly requested a foot massage from her nurse, especially when she felt weak or despairing, since it supported her will to recover.

THERAPEUTIC TOUCH

Age: Birth and older
Pain: Anxiety, restlessness, fatigue, persistent draining pain and discomfort
Time: As needed

Therapeutic touch has recently become popular as a gentle method of increasing a person's sense of peace and harmony, while easing pain and distress. It was developed 22 years ago by Dr. Dolores Krieger, professor of nursing at New York University, specifically for people working in health care, as an extension of their professional skills. It is based on the assumption that, physically, human beings are "open energy systems" and that the transfer of energy between people is thus a natural, continuous event. The therapeutic touch practitioner first focuses on the intent to help, soothe, or relax the other person and then strokes on or very close to the patient's body in even, continuous movements.

Therapeutic touch has gained popularity among nurses as a way of balancing the stress of "doing to" patients with compassionate caring for patients in pain and discomfort. Courses are offered to professionals, patients, and families in many cities throughout North America. Health professionals trained in therapeutic touch use it with children and adults suffering from chronic illnesses, such as cancer and AIDS. It soothes anxiety and induces relaxation, thus reducing pain or making it easier to handle. As a therapy, it can be used on its own, but in situations of pain it can easily be combined with analgesic medication.

ICE

Age: Six months and older
Pain: Pain related to acute injury with no open wound, bruising,
 or muscle sprains
Time: As long as needed before skin becomes numb, or maximum of 15 minutes

Ice is the cheapest and safest form of treatment to use immediately after sustaining bruises, tearing ligaments, spraining a wrist or ankle, pulling a muscle, or being bitten by an insect. It is also effective as a mild local anesthetic; the cooling effect of the ice reduces the conduction of pain signals. Cooling is especially beneficial when combined with mild to moderate pressure, such as firm application of a tensor bandage. Cooling and compression together slow blood flow and reduce muscle spasm and inflammation, limiting tissue damage and thus speeding the healing process. Above all, the sensation of coolness on a recent injury feels good.

Sports physicians usually recommend applying a compression bandage and icing an injury, a swelling, or a chronic recurring muscle or tendon pain for up to 10 to 15 minutes every hour for the first 24 to 48 hours, or until the inflammation has subsided. Physiotherapists recommend giving the injured site a 10-minute ice massage and then wrapping and, if possible, elevating the injured part. Resting and elevating the painful limb seem to help reduce inflammation and bleeding.

Children are tolerant of cold for brief periods and say that ice soothes immediate, sharp pain. Be cautious when using ice with babies under the age of six months, since they are much more sensitive and susceptible to cold and ice than older children. Some very general guidelines for using ice are listed below; it is best to first discuss with your doctor how you wish to use ice following any injury.

How to use ice

You can use ice cubes or shaved or crushed ice wrapped in a thin towel; frozen peas or corn in a plastic bag, also wrapped in a thin towel; or gel ice packs, which can be bought from the pharmacy.

- Frozen corn or peas in a plastic bag wrapped in a towel have a distinct advantage over ice, since they conform much more easily to the shape of the injured area and are convenient for traveling, should you need to take your child to the hospital.
- Be especially cautious with gel packs, which contain refreezable chemical gels that may become colder than ice and cause frostbite. Ensure that there is no puncture in the pack, since the chemicals can burn.
- To help make icing more fun, you can use commercially available gel cubes in terry cloth shapes, such as the Ouch Mouse distributed by Discovery Toys.
- Alternatively, you can cut colored sponges into favorite animal shapes, soak them in water, and freeze them. Store these in the freezer for easy access when minor accidents, bruises, and bumps occur at home. You can then give the child a choice: "You've bumped yourself! Do you want a cold bunny or a freezing giraffe to help the pain go?"

Warnings

- Do not use ice on an open or bleeding wound. Do not use ice if the child is in shock and is shivering and cold.
- Do not use ice directly on the skin. Wrap the ice in a towel, or tea towel, so that it doesn't burn the child's skin, cause frostbite, or damage nerves.
- Do not use ice for longer than ten minutes on one place, and monitor its effects every five minutes.
- Do not use ice if your child is hypersensitive to cold, has any circulatory problems, or lacks normal skin sensation.

WATER

Age: Birth and older
Pain: Pain related to mild burns, acute injury with open wound, or bruising
Time: As long as needed

Running cool water over a scraped limb serves several purposes. It cleans the wound of debris, it cools the burning pain that often accompanies the injury, and the feeling and sound of the water can be soothing for children. Cool water is also an effective first treatment for mild burns, but not for third-degree burns, where the skin has been burned off and the underlying tissue is visible. These burns require prompt medical attention.

A cool cloth is often very soothing for a child who has a headache or is feverish and achy. The child should lie down, with eyes closed, in a quiet room. Soak the cloth in cold water, wring it out, and then place it over the child's forehead.

HEAT

Age: Six months and older
Pain: Achy persistent muscle or stomach pain, pain related to acute injury with closed wounds, bruising, sprains, or muscle strains, and "growing pains"
Time: As long as it helps and feels good

Heat in the form of a heating pad, water bottle, bath or shower helps relieve pain, reduce joint stiffness, relax muscles, and ease spasms. Using heat increases the blood flow to the painful area and helps disperse the build-up of muscle waste products. Heat is very soothing for abdominal pains, menstrual cramps, and general muscle aches, since it encourages relaxation. *A precaution*: Since heat increases the blood flow, it can dislodge a newly formed blood clot that is repairing after injury, causing bleeding to recur. *A heating pad* should not be left on a child unattended; its effects should be monitored every five minutes.

A warm water bottle provides comfort that can be managed by the child, who can move it around her body onto achy muscles or menstrual pains, and the warmth relaxes spasms and provides some relief.

Warm baths are very helpful for children with achy musculoskeletal pains, fibromyalgia, or rheumatoid arthritis. The heat of the bath relaxes muscles, although if it is too hot, the bath might induce fatigue. Warm baths are often best just before bed, except for children with arthritic conditions and stiff joints. For these children, a warm bath in the morning and the evening can help mobilize joints and reduce the ache.

Warm showers with hot or warm water running or pulsing over a standing or sitting child's head eases some of the build-up of tension and muscular pain associated with tension headaches.

Michel is a 17-year-old six-footer with intermittent severe tension headaches that wipe him out for a day. He found that his severe headaches made concentrating and keeping up with school difficult. His smoking and occasional drinking added to his feelings of physical discomfort; he would feel the tension build up in his neck muscles and become "like a tight band" across his head. He occasionally resorted to smoking marijuana to alleviate the pain, but this was not effective. In fact, the resulting lack of motivation and lassitude only added to his difficulty in picking up his life again after each episode of headaches. He was willing to try other options, physical and pharmacological, in his pain-management program.

Whenever he felt the headache tension beginning, Michel immediately took two extra-strength Tylenols and would massage his neck and temples while standing in a shower, as the natural soothing action of warm, cascading water washed his tension away. (He mentioned that his showers became lengthy events.) Afterward, he would lie down and rest. By altering his posture, he could release the various strains and tensions in the muscles of his neck and head. This ritual brought his headaches from a rating of seven or eight out of ten down to a three or two within half an hour. The combination of physical strategies was just a beginning, but it was a crucial first step in enabling Michel to get a grip on the headaches that had gripped him.

ICE AND HEAT

Age: Six months and older
Pain: Painful and inflamed injury, a muscle spasm, or sore joints
Time: As long as it relieves the pain

Alternating ice and heat promotes pain relief; the ice tends to reduce inflammation, and the heat eases the muscular pain and tension. This technique works by alternating constriction and dilatation of blood vessels and acts as a mild analgesic. Using both ice and heat can be very effective for a child's sore joints. For small joints, such as finger joints, apply cold for 15 seconds, followed by warmth for 45 seconds; repeat for 10 minutes. For larger joints, such as elbow or knee, apply cold for one minute, followed by heat for one minute. Your physician's guidance is important to ensure that these methods will aid in healing your child's particular pain condition. For children with cancer or nerve damage (neuropathy), conditions in which nerve fibers are not reliable in communicating pain, you must use extra caution and frequently check the skin to prevent burns or frostbite.

ACUPUNCTURE

Age: All ages
Pain: Musculoskeletal and persistent, chronic pain
Time: Determined by a trained acupuncturist

Acupuncture has been developed and practiced in China for more than 5,000 years to relieve many medical conditions, including pain. Special fine needles are inserted through the skin into underlying tissue at strategic sites on the body known as acupuncture points. With younger children a laser is often used instead of needles—or, if laser is not available, the needles are very briefly inserted and then removed. In this practice the body is viewed as a dynamic system of organs connected by the flow of Qi (vital energy) within a complex system of hypothesized energy lines in the body known as meridians. Pain and illness result from the improper flow and balance of Qi along the meridians. Proper flow may be restored by needling or manually twirling needles in specified and established combinations of the 365 classical acupuncture points. Today acupuncture is used in the West to create analgesia for persistent pain or anesthesia for surgery, either as an adjunct to existing therapies or in some cases as the sole treatment.

Acupuncture therapy in the hands of trained acupuncturists is generally acknowledged to be a safe and effective way of treating pain, and the insertion of needles should not necessarily be painful. Not much literature exists about its use with children in pain, however. For children experiencing episodes of mild acute pain, such as dental pain, the pain and anxiety resulting from the insertion of needles may be worse than the dental pain itself. For severe or recurrent acute pain, however, such as migraine headaches that last for hours or days, acupuncture may be beneficial. It is not yet clearly understood how acupuncture relieves pain. It is thought to work through the central (not the peripheral) nervous system by activating the body's own pain-inhibiting system, which either raises the pain threshold or modulates the response to pain. Used widely with adults suffering from chronic pain, acupuncture may be easier for teenagers to handle than for younger children, unless a laser, which is totally painless, is used for treatment.

ACUPRESSURE

Age: One year and older
Pain: Headaches, dental pain, shoulder and back pain
Time: Brief and as required (can be repeated every two to three hours) or as determined by a physiotherapist or massage therapist

Acupressure is derived from acupuncture. Specific points are stimulated not by acupuncture but by finger pressure or rubbing. One of the most powerful analgesic points is known as Hoku, a highly sensitive acupuncture point located in the web of skin in the muscle between the thumb and forefinger. Hoku, also known as Large Intestine 4 because it is on the large intestine meridian, is the second most important point in acupuncture. For tension headaches or dental pain, strong (and not always pleasant) pressure is delivered to the point with finger or thumb on both hands for 30 to 40 seconds; this procedure can be repeated every two to three hours. When the point is stimulated correctly, a red ring, which is associated with endorphin release, appears around it. Pressure on the point can be painful, but the subsequent pain relief in the other areas can be quite marked. When combined with pressure on additional points identified by an acupuncturist, physiotherapist, or massage therapist as helpful to a specific pain, the analgesic effects for the child or teen can be enhanced.

TENS*

Age: Three years and older
Pain: Various pains, including burn pain, muscle aches and spasms, incision pain, bone metastasis, neuropathy, shingles, phantom limb pains
Time: 30 minutes, two to three times per day, or as advised

Traditionally TENS (transcutaneous electrical nerve stimulation) has been viewed as a device to relieve muscle pains and pain from surgery incisions; however, it also relieves pain associated with headaches, burns, damaged nerves, the spread of cancer to ribs and other bones, phantom limb pain, painful intravenous inserts (IVs), intramuscular injections, arthritis, and painful wounds. Precautions need to be taken for people who have epilepsy or cardiac problems. Although TENS can be used on its own for pain relief, it combines well with other pain-relieving methods.

---

* The sections on TENS and acupressure were written with Dr. Jo Eland, associate professor of nursing at The University of Iowa. Dr. Eland has extensive experience in the use of these methods and has pioneered the use of TENS with children.

What is TENS?

TENS units are battery-powered, pager-sized plastic boxes, with attached wires and electrodes, which are placed on selected sites on a patient's body. The unit delivers electrical impulses through the surface of the skin via black rubber electrodes, which are attached to the skin's surface with gels and karaya. The electrodes come in many shapes and sizes, and most can be cut with scissors to fit a specific body part, a property that makes it useful for children's smaller bodies. Three types of TENS can be selected: conventional, brief intense, and acupuncture-like. Each type has several settings that can be modified to improve pain control. Children tend not to like acupuncture-like TENS and to better tolerate the brief intense TENS and conventional TENS.

How does TENS work?

TENS transmits electrical impulses along the nerves competing with the pain messages and thereby acting as pain inhibitors. In addition, the stimulation helps the brain release endorphins, our naturally occurring form of morphine. How can electricity, which is not benign, be helpful in relieving pain? Most people have rightfully regarded the use of electricity to relieve pain with caution. The amount of energy delivered through the TENS electrodes, however, is very small. In fact, every time your heart beats it puts out more electricity than a TENS unit.

Most TENS units have three basic controls that can be selected and adjusted by the person in pain: rate, pulse width, and amplitude.

- The rate determines the number of electrical impulses delivered through the skin. A low rate is experienced as a pulse; a faster rate, as vibrations.
- The pulse width, or the duration of the pulse, controls how deeply the pain-relieving signal goes into the tissue. A low pulse width keeps the electrical sensation on the surface of the skin, which is helpful in relieving the pain of wounds, such as an incision or skin lesion. A higher pulse width sends the signal more deeply into the tissue.
- The amplitude settings are highly individualized, controlling how many milliamps are delivered to the skin surface. Children and families have to experiment with the settings to determine which are most pleasant and provide the greatest pain relief. The amplitude should be turned up in order to create a strong pleasant sensation. It is incorrect to think that a higher number on the amplitude is better

for relieving pain than a lower amplitude, however. TENS should *never* cause pain or make existing pain worse.

- Additional controls can provide a massage-like sensation or alternate six seconds of the electrical signal with a six-second pause. This latter use is thought to prevent the area from becoming accustomed to the stimulation, an important factor for relieving some types of pain.

Sixteen-year-old Enrico was driving home one day when a car ran a stop sign in front of him, causing him to smash into the side of an old pick-up truck. In the sudden impact, he sustained a concussion, and in the emergency room, it was discovered that his retina was also significantly detached. He had a variety of treatments, including laser therapy. As a result of the injury, however, his trigeminal nerve (the nerve that supplies the forehead, upper cheek, and eye) had become terribly bruised. This pain was hot stabbing (neuropathic) pain; his eye hurt terribly, and he was seeing double and feeling quite desperate. It was difficult to control the pain of his damaged nerve using medication, so the nurse recommended trying TENS. One electrode was placed above his eye and one below, and with the controls in his own hands, he adjusted them to a pulse that felt good. After 15 minutes of continual TENS, he was pain-free. TENS became Enrico's primary method of pain control for the following year until he had healed enough not to have to use it regularly.

TENS can help minimize or relieve many types of pain, even short-term needle pain, when other alternatives don't work or are not available.

Amy, aged four, had leukemia. As part of her treatment, she had to have an intramuscular injection every day for six weeks. The injection of chemotherapy hurt, so Amy and her parents were keen to use anything that would help. Since topical anesthetic solutions were not yet available at their clinic, they chose a TENS unit. Every morning after breakfast Amy's mother put the TENS unit on her daughter. One electrode went across Amy's leg above the knee cap and the other up her leg at her panty line. With the unit working, Amy watched her favorite TV show, "Reading Rainbow," after which she and her mother went to the clinic with the TENS unit still on and working. After two days Amy became so at ease with the routine that she would skip down the hall to the treatment room ahead of her mother and allow the nurse to give the injection. Only then did Amy take the TENS unit off, handing it to her mom. With her pain well controlled, Amy no longer had to be carried, clinging and crying, from her house to the car to the clinic. Instead she became willing to make the injection part of her daily routine.

Benefits of TENS for children

Since TENS has been used mostly with adults, there is little information about using TENS with children. This dearth of data is unfortunate, for TENS has many features that are highly desirable for children: in particular, it is non-invasive (requires no needles), it is a neat little device that a school-aged child can apply and control, and it provides fairly steady reduction in or relief from pain. Adult research has shown that for a longer-lasting analgesic effect, TENS should be applied for at least 30 minutes. This time must be individually adjusted to the child and the type of pain. For example, to control pain during burn treatment, TENS is used for 5 to 15 minutes.

CARRYING, RAPID ROCKING, AND SUCKING A PACIFIER

Age: Birth to one year
Pain: Sudden minor pain or distress, heelsticks, immunizations, colic, and incessant crying
Time: 5 to 10 minutes

We know that close body contact and being carried reduces an infant's crying. A baby is soothed when swaddled and held or carried in a pouch close to a parent's body. Sucking a pacifier, the breast, or a bottle regulates the infant's breathing and often enables an infant to settle when distressed or in pain. The combination of being swaddled, moving, sucking, and hearing a familiar voice provides comfort for newborns and babies in their first year of life.

If very distressed, an infant that has colic or that is incessantly crying after a minor medical procedure can be swaddled, held, and rapidly rocked (50 beats or more per minute). With the infant's or baby's head well supported, rapid rocking can be combined with rhythmic patting, and the regulated rhythm will bring the crying baby's distressed and disorganized respiration into an almost synchronistic pattern. Used in this way, rapid rocking sets a regular pace that guides the baby's erratic crying breaths into a more settled pattern. Large, smooth movements, rather than tight, abrupt ones, create a steady, powerful pattern that soothes both child and caregiver, especially if they are combined with rhythmic singing. It is most effective when a young baby is crying incessantly or seems fatigued, or when colic has been diagnosed. This method requires energy but, sometimes after five to ten minutes of rapid rocking, the baby will fall asleep. It is usually as effective at soothing an infant as the sound of a vacuum cleaner and is safer than a drive in the car!

Some early findings suggest that a drop of sugar or glucose water on the newborn baby's tongue before a heelstick blood test reduces the amount of crying following this procedure. The findings indicate that the effect of sugar water may be best at two to three days after birth and disappears over the first six months of life. Before an infant receives an immunization, pre-empt the pain by giving the infant a recommended dose of acetaminophen one hour before the injection, then provide the baby with a pacifier dipped in sugar water to suck a few minutes before the needle and allow the baby to vigorously suck through and after the procedure. For invasive procedures, EMLA (see p. 178), a local anesthetic in cream form, is available by prescription for children six months and over. All these simple methods—swaddling, carrying, rocking, patting, and allowing the baby to suck a pacifier dipped in sugar water, or to suck from the breast—are safe and helpful soothing methods for infants in their first year of life.

BREATHING METHODS

Have you noticed how your breathing changes when you are feeling angry or afraid? You may take deep, trembling breaths when you are angry or hold your breath when you are afraid. How you feel immediately affects your breathing. The reverse is also true; breathing affects how you feel and behave, as many practitioners of the martial arts, actors, and other performers well know. By changing breathing patterns, the karate practitioner is able to concentrate, focus energy, and change fear into effective action. Physiological states, metabolism rate, heart rate, respiration rate, perspiration, and blood pressure all change as a function of controlled breathing. Breathing has a profound effect on our physical and psychological functioning. In essence, it is a crucial link between mind and body.

The physiological benefits of breathing

Each time a deep, long breath is drawn into the body, a number of very important physical changes occur in the spine, the diaphragm, the rib cage, and even the stomach. With a deep breath, the lungs expand, gently stretching the vertebrae in the upper spinal column. As the lungs expand, the diaphragm flattens out, massaging the stomach. At the same time as the breath fills the lungs, the muscles between the ribs expand horizontally, stretching the back and torso of the body. The increase in oxygen in the body produces a feeling of well-being.

Despite the beneficial effect of breathing deeply, our instinctive reaction when in pain is to still our breath so as not to cause any more pain by deep breathing. This is a protective reaction, but it does not relieve the pain. When breathing is shut down in this manner, contraction in the muscle fiber increases and tension builds. In contrast, each time you exhale, you release muscle tension and rigidity, and pain can disperse. With a series of generous, deep exhalations, the resulting neuromuscular release increases relaxation, eases pain, and releases pressure on the sensory nervous system in those muscles.

If this release does not occur and the muscles remain protective, overactive, and tense around the pain site, neuromuscular fatigue continually builds up and increases, heightening the pain. Worse, over time the neuromuscular pathways begin to confuse the messages of pain and tension so that they become intertwined, and a vicious cycle of pain, tension, and fatigue continues to escalate. Since pain and anxiety are intertwined, mastering your breath during pain controls anxiety as well.

Exhalation is the key to breaking the pain cycle; it is best to start by exhaling forcefully. By first emptying the lungs, you can get fresh air to enter. Breathing in a *regular, easy rhythm* releases pain. This rhythmic action is comforting and predictable, like a regular heart beat, and so everything else can fall into a normal pattern. Protective fear, the need to hold tight, falls away. Rhythmic breathing can be a valuable asset when pain, distress, or anxiety is a part of your life.*

Learning to recognize, regulate, and manage breathing is surprisingly easy for children. Those who are school aged and older, in particular, find this mastery rewarding to use whenever they are in pain. The use of breathing methods can bolster their self-confidence and feelings of self-worth, as well as lessening the pain and distress. Following is a description of breathing techniques that can be used for toddlers, children, and teenagers.

Blowing Away the Pain

Age: One year and older
Pain: Acute, brief pain, from scrapes, falls, or injections, anticipatory anxiety, persistent achy pain, abdominal or limb pain, disease-related pain, and pain associated with medical treatments

---

* People with lung problems, such as asthma, people with post-polio syndrome, or people with lung disease will tell you that the instantaneous effect of not being able to exhale, to release their breath, or to inhale enough air into their lungs causes profound anxiety. Theirs is not a mental anxiety but a bodily reaction, a physiological panic resulting from insufficient air throughout their system.

Time: Two to ten minutes, or for the duration of the pain

When you exhale, as if you're blowing the candles out, your lungs empty and then you automatically inhale. Regulated breathing expands the ribs and spine and stretches muscles, easing tension and allowing pain and discomfort to be released. Tell the child to "blow out the pain" and demonstrate, blowing out a steady slow breath. Then blow out with the child, ensuring that the child does not hyperventilate, but blows steadily, thinking about the pain leaving his body.

This simple method can be used for many types of pain and can be taught to children from one year of age and up. (Although some people are surprised that a year-old toddler would know how to blow, remember that a one-year-old adores blowing out candles.) Toddlers and younger children depend heavily on their parents' involvement in engaging and sustaining breathing techniques. Keep in mind that your attitude and support will make or break the successful application of this method.

Children aged six and older can usually regulate breathing by themselves. Children with recurrent pain report that blowing away the pain when their pain recurs helps both to settle pain and contain anxiety. Other children say that blowing on a scrape helps to cool the pain. This breathing method is extremely useful during procedures that require the child to remain still for two to ten minutes, such as receiving an injection, having an IV inserted, having lacerations stitched, or having a cast placed on a fractured bone, as well as during less traumatic procedures, such as having an X-ray, a bone scan, or other medical assessment procedures. To be sure, pain medication is often given to the child, but until it takes effect, blowing away the pain can settle the child and even increase the effectiveness of the medication. Breathing gives the child something helpful to do while the procedure takes place, since being still is not a natural state for most awake children!

Nine-year-old Seanna had mastered blowing out as her preferred way of ridding herself of scary feelings and distress before and during spinal taps, part of the treatment for her leukemia. She feared that after she was discharged from hospital she might forget how to do her blowing, her mainstay. So she practiced regularly, taking little chunks of time out of her day, in case she had to return into hospital. This example speaks of her determination: whenever her mother went to the supermarket, she would stay in the car and practice her blowing!

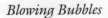

Blowing Bubbles

Age: One year and older
Pain: Acute, brief pain, as from a scrape, fall, injections, or IV starts
Time: Before and for the duration of the pain

Bubbles, party blowers, pinwheels, and similar devices can sustain a child's regular breathing to relieve pain and anxiety while adding an element of fun. Children like to blow colorful bubbles of different sizes and watch them travel across the room. They also like to respond to an inviting challenge in an otherwise anxious or uncertain situation. For example: "See how far you can blow this bubble," "I wonder how many twin bubbles you will blow this time while I look at your veins," or "Can you catch a bubble and blow even more bubbles from it while I wash your skin clean? I wonder how many more it'll make." Throughout this purposeful activity, instead of being gripped by fear and pain, the child begins to feel the sweet sense of success and competence while controlling anxiety or pain.

Remember that most children regress when they are in pain. We have thus found bubble blowing to be an effective method with a wide age range, from one to ten years of age. Children are individuals. Some children become totally absorbed in the task and the relief that bubble blowing provides and continue blowing long after the acute pain has ceased. Some may refuse to blow, may reject the bubble wand, or choose to blow out without bubbles. It is the child's pain, and the child should decide what works and how to participate in the process. Thus, the coach need not feel defeated and throw the method out just because it hasn't worked on the first occasion. At the next procedure the child may surprise everyone by spontaneously blowing or requesting the bubbles. Give the child the opportunity to learn and to choose the method she wants.

BREATHING-RELAXATION METHOD

Age: Seven years and older
Pain: Non-acute, persistent achy pain, abdominal or limb pain, and disease-related pain such as Crohn's disease, and syndromes such as irritable bowel and chronic fatigue.
Time: 10 to 30 minutes

For older children and teens, breathing techniques can easily be combined with lying down, closing one's eyes, and letting go. Children know and enjoy this state; for example, 12-year-old Kevin relaxed by becoming a wet noodle! Once begun, the relaxation process will lead the child into a gradually deepening state of repose characterized by increasing feelings of warmth and comfort. Many physiological changes naturally occur when one is relaxing. Pain, such as abdominal or bowel pain, and achy muscles and ligaments may soften and ease as the exercise progresses. Relaxation should never be used as a substitute for taking needed pain relief medication, but when combined with an analgesic, breathing relaxation significantly relieves anxiety and pain.

Most school-aged children can become proficient using relaxation and breathing methods, independently of an adult. Children with persistent or recurrent pain find that 10 to 15 minutes of daily or regular practice of breathing relaxation or relaxation combined with imagery (see later in this chapter) has long-term benefits. During treatment, I regularly make children their own relaxation imagery audio tape for use at home on a cassette player or Walkman.

Younger children, in contrast, find the concept of relaxing difficult to grasp. Some associate relaxing with sleep—something children want to avoid. Since children under six sometimes even find it hard to keep their eyes closed, if you wish to do a relaxation exercise with them, focus their eyes on something in the room. Younger children in pain respond positively to a more lively process, such as interacting with the telling of their favorite stories, rather than the slow, calming process of relaxing. Don't be perturbed by wriggling or movement; it doesn't mean that the child isn't attending to or absorbing your words but rather that younger children often reveal their thinking by movement and play.

Do some of these relaxation and imagery exercises yourself so that you can better appreciate the process when you do it with a child. First:

- Ensure that you will not be interrupted. Put a sign on the door that warns, "Work in progress" or "Do not disturb," and unplug the telephone.
- Ensure that both you and your child are comfortable: Your child should lie on her back, if possible, on a couch or bed, without crossing her legs or arms. You need to feel as easy and relaxed as possible so that you can convey this calm and comfort in your voice, pacing, focus, and style.
- Ensure that your child is warm, preferably covered by a light blanket, since warmth promotes muscle relaxation, and loosen any belt or tight clothing.

Talking slowly and calmly, guide the child through breathing relaxation, by instructing the child in this way:

Make yourself as comfortable as you can be . . . let all of your breath out of your body . . . now it's easy to let your lungs fill up all by themselves. Notice how your lungs know exactly how much air to take in, how long to hold, and how to automatically let your breath out. Follow your breath; you follow it. Track how each breath has its own timing and rhythm—your body knows how to breathe automatically. Keep your attention following your breath and observe how your breath breathes your body. It's an effortless, natural, easy, wonderful process.

Notice also, with your attention on your breath, how the tension is beginning to go out of your body. Your muscles release, becoming softer, looser, more and more comfortable. Notice how some parts of your body may feel heavier and other parts may feel lighter—it's very interesting. Notice it all. Notice how your body is becoming warmer and pleasant sensations are getting stronger. You may notice that one part of your body is feeling particularly warm and that another part, maybe your arms, feels particularly heavy. Another part, I'm not sure which, feels very good. It's so nice to just let go and go with the flow of your breath, as the relaxation eases your pain farther and farther away.

Breathing relaxation uses the focus on breath to lead the child into greater relaxation. There are other ways of achieving relaxation:

Relaxing from toes to top Focus attention systematically on each part of the body, starting from the tips of the child's toes, inviting the child to release any tension from each part of the body as you gradually work up to the crown of the head. (Alternatively you can start with the head and progress down to the toes.)

Counting breaths This activity deepens breathing in a controlled way, quickening the relaxation effect. The counts can be stated aloud or the child can count inwardly, while lying down with eyes closed. The key is to breathe rhythmically in the following way: count to three for an exhalation, suspend breathing for the count of three, then inhale for the count of three, and hold the breath for a count of three (3x3x3x3). Repeat this cycle and, as the breathing slows, you can move to a counting cycle of four, that is, 4x4x4x4. As you progress, it can induce sleep. Generally, this relaxation variant is more suited to older children and teenagers than to children ten and younger.

Practice progressive relaxation Certain muscles in the limbs and trunk can be selectively tensed and then released. Children who are not aware of carrying tension in their muscles or who have trouble relaxing find this method beneficial. Here is the way to guide a child through the process:

Lying down comfortably, close your eyes and let your breath out fully. Take a deep breath in and exhale slowly. With all your muscles as relaxed as they can possibly be, focus all your attention on your right arm. Squeeze your right hand into a fist, hold it tight for the count of five, and now relax it. Feel the difference in your hand. Now bend your arm, making a muscle, hold it tight for five seconds, and relax it completely. Feel the change in sensation and comfort and notice what has changed. Push your arm into the bed, feel the tension, hold it for five seconds, and let it go. Enjoy the release as your arm relaxes fully into the bed. Pay attention to how your whole arm feels now and how different the other arm feels. (Repeat this process on the left side. You can follow this with tensing and relaxing the toes, feet, calves, and thighs on one leg, drawing the child's attention to changes in sensation, and then repeat with the other limb.)

Whatever permutation or creative variation of relaxation you develop with your child, the more frequently it is practiced, the more quickly the child will derive positive results.

IMAGERY METHODS

Imagery is the spontaneous or deliberate mental reconstruction of sights, sounds, smells, tastes, and feelings as if they were actually occurring. As part of our inner life, images carry personal meaning and power and undoubtedly play a central role in helping the body heal. Imagery generates new internal experiences, and thus is an active process, unlike the passive act of relaxing or ingesting medication. Whether they spontaneously spring to mind or are consciously created, images help to bring a desirable state closer to reality. Focusing on chosen or favorite images provides an opportunity to escape from pain and not be preoccupied with it. Even more important, focusing on *altering* the image or sensations of the pain may enable a child in pain to gain more control over and relief from the pain. Imagery needs to be gentle, child-centered, and energy conserving to relieve children's and adolescents' pain and suffering.

About imagery with children

Imagining is a spontaneous and natural act for children. In fact, children think in images and learn to recognize objects in the world using all of their senses. Most children imagine primarily in pictures or sounds, whereas fewer experience body sensation or smells. A child's primary sense may be vision; nevertheless, all other senses can be called upon to reconstruct a memory or to create a new vision. Here are some directions that lead the child to use each of the senses:

Visual: "I wonder what you can see."

Auditory: "Listen to what sounds are here." Olfactory: "I wonder what
   smell you may notice that you really like." Gustatory: "There may be a
   taste there too; what does it remind you of?"

Touch: "What can you touch or feel in your body right now?"

Imagery is also a specific method for producing physiological
changes. "The images we spin inwardly become the reality we spin out,"
writes Maureen Murdock in her lovely book on imagery with children,
Spinning Inward, a fine resource on guided imagery with children. As
the child's absorption in the imagery increases, the capacity to increase
comfort, dissociate from the pain, reduce anxiety, or alter the discomfort becomes greater.

Children's images are unique and unexpected and vary from child to
child. Work with images that your child prefers and avoid disliked experiences. For example, if the child is afraid of the water, the thought of
"swimming with the fishes" is unlikely to promote relief, whereas re-
creating an activity that she adores is more likely to provide the necessary relief. Use the child's own spontaneous images, such as sitting on
the sun to increase body temperature, rather than your own or more
standard images. If imagery is started when pain first enters a child's life
and is regularly used, it becomes a reliable source of support and
strength for a child in intermittent or chronic pain.

Some children may be reluctant at first to become involved in imagery exercises and may put up some resistance. Be flexible and don't
push. You could say that imagery often helps the pain to ease and that
you're curious about how it will help. If your child isn't interested, let it
go. It is not the right time or the right method for your child. Resistance
may be a sign that having an outside professional as coach may be what
the child needs to learn effective methods of pain relief. Monitor the
child's facial expressions, position, and movements; these indicate the
child's degree of involvement with the imagery and whether it is providing relief. If you note that something is amiss, you can ask: "What's
happening?" Supportive dialogue can sometimes enhance the effectiveness of the imagery. The child will sense that support and enter the experience more fully to obtain relief.

You can construct an imagery experience in two ways. First, invite
the child or teen to choose a favorite person, place, activity, or story. Focus on creating a rich experience with the child that uses all the senses.

When the present reality is fraught with pain, anxiety, fear, and tension, this focus helps the child to distance himself from the pain and sometimes even escape it. The imagery is experienced as either leaving the pain behind or replacing it with a familiar activity or a favorite story. Second, if the pain isn't overwhelming, suggest that the child or teen focus on generating a direct image of the pain, such as a red ball of fire, then altering, shrinking, or changing it to decrease the hurting and discomfort. These imagery methods are described in greater detail below.

Leaving the pain behind

Age: Five and older
Pain: Persistent pain
Time: 5 to 25 minutes

Some children like imagining that they are going to a favorite place, and for many that place is the beach. Ten-year-old Margareta would go to the sea, where the rhythms of the waves, like her breath, allowed the pain in her tummy to settle like the sand at the bottom of the ocean. Margareta found the pain would subside quite rapidly, despite the fact that on one occasion, to her distress, she had envisioned herself on the beach with no swimsuit on!

To encourage the images that you and your child generate to flow into a helpful experience, invite your child to settle into a comfortable position and quietly say:

Close your eyes, because then you can experience everything more clearly. Let your breath out now, as your body settles down . . . down into this pink fluffy cloud, soft, yet strong enough to lift you up, up, and away from your bed, your pain, and your discomfort. Everything you don't want remains down below—your aches, your cast, the pain—as your body is lifted up, up in the sky. The wind gently lifts the cloud and you float effortlessly and rapidly across the sky, faster than any car or train taking you to Disneyland/Candyland/a grandparent's home/a holiday spot. Isn't it wonderful to notice how the closer you get to this place, the farther away you are from that discomfort. You can probably notice it getting farther and fainter and smaller, so it doesn't bother you anymore. You just snuggle into the pink cloud, pulling it over you like a blanket, feeling warm and good. Here we come . . . I wonder what you see first . . . and what you smell [use the five senses to elaborate the experience for the child]. What would you like to do here? [Create a pleasurable, fun, playful experience together. If possible, allow the child to tell you what the experience would be.] Soon it will be time to leave, but it's so good to know that we can come back here again, and so easily. When we reach your room, you may be surprised to notice that while we were gone the discomfort dissolved a little, or a lot, so that when you open your eyes, you'll be feeling pretty good, filled with memories of [this place] and wonderful good feelings in your body.

How much the pain decreases will vary, depending on the child's ability to imagine an alternative experience that creates distance from the pain. Older children and teens can be enormously inventive in using images to change the perception of their pain.

Seventeen-year-old Jason found one simple image that could always be counted on to help him deal with the gnawing abdominal pain from the recurring ulcerative colitis constriction in his colon. His method combined distancing himself from the pain and altering it. Concentrating, he imagined all his pain being put into a bag, similar to an intravenous bag that carries fluids and hangs from an IV pole. When he had stuffed all his pain into the bag, he would deliberately imagine taking the bag and hanging it on the far side of the IV pole, a distance away from the bed in which he lay. He would repeat this one-minute exercise whenever he needed to, with a certain mischievous glee, as he hung his pain out of his body.

Replacing pain with a familiar activity

Age: 5 and older
Pain: Persistant pain
Time: as long as needed

Replacing the pain is a variation on "leaving the pain behind"; the pain is replaced by an engrossing activity that leaves no room for pain. Older children and teens can readily relive a favorite activity that they do regularly. Activities like skating, swimming, cycling, playing soccer, and skiing, or quieter activities like reading a book, listening to music, sorting football or hockey cards, or playing with dolls can be easily harnessed to become an absorbing, fun-filled reality to replace the experience of pain.

Kim, a keen sportsman, was diagnosed at 13 years of age with Crohn's disease, a disease of the small intestine. He experienced severe crampy abdominal pain and diarrhea. Since he enjoyed physical activity, when his pains began he drew on images from his sports career to help him through the painful crampy spasms that characterize this disease. He would focus on becoming as comfortable as possible, though that was often hard. Then he would take himself skiing down one of his favorite runs.

In the beginning it was difficult, he said, for the pain would pull him back. But then, he told me, he would focus on the powdery snow, the sound of his skiis making tracks where no one else had been. He would focus on moving, on his crouched position as he prepared to fly over a mogul, twisting and turning, and on the feeling in his legs. Then he would focus on the sights: the sun peering through the alpine trees heavy with snow, the village so small in the valley below. If this was difficult, he would conjure up smells: the crisp winter air, the smell of wet snow. He would come to the end of his run, sometimes five to seven minutes later, filled with energy and free of pain for a while.

The effect of imagery can last longer than the actual imagery experience.

Telling Favorite Stories
Age: Two to six years
Pain: Any mild, moderate persisting or treatment-related pain
Time: 5 to 15 minutes

Young children's favorite stories have a particular power. Often children will ask to have their favorite story read over and over again. Children experience a delight in this ritual, in its predictability, and its associations, in anticipating what is going to happen and chiming in at the more dramatic moments. Preschoolers often know their stories by heart. As a result, these favorite stories can be very helpful to draw on during scary or painful times.

Five-year-old Samantha was referred to me for her fear of pain. I saw her before the dreaded bone marrow aspiration, a part of her cancer treatment. I asked her if she liked the story "Snow White." "I don't want that story!" she said emphatically. "I want the story of Grandma Tildy and the Elephant!" Not having heard the story, I asked her to tell it to me. She told the story vividly, complete with concrete details and sound effects. "Now how about if I tell you the story of 'Grandma Tildy and the Elephant' while your bone marrow gets done?" I suggested, "I wouldn't be surprised if, by the time we got to the end of the story, the bone marrow was over and the Band-aid was on. Wouldn't that be nice?" Samantha nodded. We had a working contract. Tightly holding her "Kitty," she anxiously walked into the surgery room and climbed onto the table. I told the staff what we had decided to do and began the story: "Grandma Tildy lived by herself and was such a brave little lady. One day there was a knock [knocking sound effects] on the door . . ." Samantha's attention was glued to the details of the story. Her body moved when the sensations were uncomfortable, but her eyes were fixed and her concentration did not waver. I stretched out the details and increased the inten-

sity and excitement of the story during the more painful parts of the medical pro-
cedure so that the story remained competitive with her discomfort.

After the procedure, Samantha told me that the pain was a five out of five,
but her scary feelings were only a one out of five. This discrepancy suggested that
Samantha continued to be aware of the pain of the procedure, despite the local
anesthetic, but in contrast to previous occasions, when she would cry, this time the
procedure did not bother her much.

Sometimes with focused concentration and absorption in something like a favorite story, pain sensations may not be entirely eradicated but may simply become less relevant and therefore less upsetting and scary.

The favorite story technique, like all the methods described, needs to be tailored to each child's needs and temperament. The only way you'll know whether it fits is to let the story unfold. There is no substitute for the telling. The tales can be creatively altered to offer metaphors for courage, competence, and accomplishment during taxing times. Many of the classic fairy tales easily lend themselves to this, for they powerfully evoke previous associations of coping and memories of comfort and security, and many fairy tales themselves are about enduring trials, facing challenges, and overcoming overwhelming difficulties.

Shrinking the pain

Age: Five years and older
Pain: Any mild or moderate persistent pain
Time: 5 to 15 minutes

With regular practice, shrinking the pain helps the child generate inner strength and greater self-reliance in working with pain. Adapting the language for the age of your child, you can lead your child into this imagery experience by gently saying the following:

Close your eyes and breathe out. Take in a breath and again breathe out, releasing
all tension. Take one final cleansing breath as you enter inside your body by what-
ever route you wish—through your nose, on your breath, or through the holes in the
pores of your skin or your ear . . . Travel all the way to your pain. See your pain . . .
Look at it from every angle—from top and bottom and each side . . . Notice what
color it is, what shape, if it is dense or not. Then take out your magnifying glass and
inspect it, choosing the area to shrink. Taking out a can of shrinking solution, spray
the solution thickly over the entire area of the pain, on the top, on the sides, and un-
derneath, doing a thorough job. Observe your pain beginning to shrink, changing
in density, becoming more porous as the solution is absorbed, and changing color as

it becomes smaller and smaller. Take out your magnifying glass and inspect it as shrinks. Give it a final spray, allowing it to shrink away as far as it can. Enjoy the lovely space you've created. Experience the difference in sense and feeling. Leave your body by the route you entered . . . and take a deep breath in. As you breathe out, notice the changes . . . and slowly open your eyes. Allow yourself to be creative.

Pain can be shrunk in many ways. Develop the possibilities with your child, assessing which works most quickly and lasts longest.

Painting the pain
Age: 5 and older
Pain: Mild, moderate, persistant
Time: 5 to 25 minutes

Painting the pain to alter the sensation is a variation on shrinking and changing the pain. Children who enjoy art enjoy this experience. The following example begins with some breathing to allow the child, whatever the nature of the pain, to become relaxed. Invite the child to become comfortable by sitting or lying down and then to take three deep breaths.

Go into Innerland and take yourself to a big painting tent. Inside you'll find an easel and a table filled with pots of paints in many different colors. Paint a picture of your body. Now choose a color that best shows the kind of pain you have and paint the pain into the picture of your body. Brush it over all of the areas where you hurt. If there are different kinds of pain, choose the color that best describes each kind of pain. You may use a lighter shade of the color for the areas that are not hurting as much and a more intense color for the areas that are hurting the most. Do a thorough job so that your picture shows exactly how your pain is. Check it out.

After you've finished, take a pail of whitewash and pour it all over your picture. Feel and watch how the whitewash gradually seeps down, washing out the intense colors, softening and making the light color even lighter. If you wish, you can pour more whitewash and experience how that soothes the pain more. Guide the wash to areas that need it most. Watch how it soaks into your body picture and changes the pain. Now you can step back from the picture of your body as the picture gets smaller and smaller. You can then lock the picture into your mind where you can recall it whenever you want to wash a new pain away.

COMBINING PAIN IMAGERY WITH MEDICATION

Imagery exercises that change pain also work well when combined with pain medications. Brain and body interact to minimize pain and suffering. The effects seem synergistic: the medications enhance the effectiveness of the imagery in altering the pain, and the brain's absorption in the imagery seems to aid the impact of the analgesic. In addition, since analgesics can take 10 to 20 minutes to be absorbed by the system, imagery is ideal to use while the medication is being absorbed.

Fifteen-year-old Jamie was having a difficult time sleeping in the hospital. Achy bone pain from her cancer tumor, IV pumps with alarms, steadily infused morphine into her system, the lights, the sounds of other children, interruptions at night, and her own highly active mind—all contributed to her discomfort and insomnia. She was wary of using imagery but agreed to discuss the possibility. After exploring several options, she agreed to listen to relaxing music to calm herself and to focus her mind and then to see what images came to her. She saw her hip as a throbbing red fireball, emitting spurts of fire down her leg and across her pelvis [this is nerve pain]. I suggested: "How about making snowballs and throwing them on the fire, one after the other?" The quenching of the pain began slowly. After about ten minutes, the combination of pain-relieving methods began to work for Jamie. The session was audio-taped for her, with the music she had chosen in the background. Jamie used the tape at times throughout her hospitalization and at home. The hospital and its noises became irrelevant, and her "achiness" eased and she would fall asleep.

HYPNOSIS

Age: Three years and older
Pain: Acute and chronic pain
Time: As needed
Note: *Hypnosis must be carried out by a qualified health professional*

Hypnosis is a valuable tool for managing many forms of pain and discomfort. Over the last 25 years it has become increasingly used and valued by health care professionals as a primary or additional pain-relief method for children and adolescents. Although we still don't know the precise neurophysiological mechanisms by which hypnosis alleviates suffering and diminishes pain, we know that it works. Hypnosis is essentially an altered state of consciousness, or a trance, which is characterized by a temporary suspension of critical judgment, rapid assimilation of information, the capacity to alter sensation and perception, and the capacity to make feelings, sensations, or ideas fit that don't usually fit. During hypnosis for pain relief, a change in the child's perception of pain is facilitated. This change appears to bypass the child's conscious effort. The practitioner invites the child to shift into an altered state of consciousness by focusing and nar-rowing his attention. Hypnosis is an experience that is more intense and more purposefully directed than imagery. The difference between hypno-sis and imagery may not be one of kind but of degree: more intense in-volvement, greater changes in sensation and perception, and the use of therapeutic suggestions used toward a therapeutic goal.

Hypnosis includes suggestions for change; these are effective only when the child or teen is in a trance state. Suggestions can take many forms; here is an example: "You'll notice within the next one minute of clock time how much the pain will diminish. It may reduce by half or by three-quarters. You can let go and notice how much of the pain goes." Being in a trance makes it possible for a child or teen to be open to rapid change in pain.

Children in a hypnotic trance can achieve analgesia and partial anes-thesia; some individuals can create complete anesthesia in selected body parts. The goal is to provide the child with some degree of control over the sensations of pain, to diminish the pain (it isn't always possible to remove pain entirely), and to release anxiety.

It is important that the hypnotic experience be guided by a suitably qualified health care professional, psychologist, physician, nurse, social worker, or child-life worker who has received training from an accred-ited institution. Be alert: many individuals who do not have the neces-sary background or training call themselves "hypnotherapists" but are not qualified to treat pain and, therefore, are not safe to consult.

Hypnosis and imagery can be combined with other methods, such as TENS or biofeedback.

BIOFEEDBACK

Age: Three years and older
Pain: Migraine and tension headaches, moderate persisting muscle pains or disease-related pain, pain caused by stress
Time: 10 to 30 minutes; practice guided by a professional improves results

Biofeedback is the monitoring and altering of a biological function usually not thought to be under voluntary control. It is a well-docu-mented and effective therapy for adults and children, and unlike other methods, it allows the child to experience objective feedback of his or her physiological functions. A body signal, such as peripheral body tem-perature, heart rate, electrical brain activity, or muscle tension, is con-tinuously fed back as a sound or in a visual form so that the child can attempt to change the signal in the desired direction, such as decreasing muscle tension. Without this feedback, the person would have no awareness of these changes. Children and teenagers are usually interested in and enthusiastic about this method and quickly learn it. Training consists of learning to recognize the body's signal and then training it to produce change. Emphasizing the child's control and development of body self-regulation, the biofeedback technique is evidence of the continual interaction of body and brain and demonstrates how emotion and stress can play a part in creating or maintaining pain.

Eighteen-year-old Jonathan, diagnosed with tension headaches that had recurred over three years, described his pain as a tight band across his forehead. A clinical assessment and interview revealed that Jonathan tended to keep quiet about matters that worried him and to avoid problems rather than deal with them directly. In conversation, Jonathan said it was unlikely that his difficulties, particularly those with a group at school, were contributing to his headache.

Since he was intrigued by the notion of biofeedback, we placed self-stick electrodes from the machine on his forehead and temples (the frontalis muscle) to monitor the tension levels as we discussed aspects of his life. This made the brain-body interaction more evident. When the muscle tension increased, the beeps got progressively faster, but when he began to relax the muscle, the beeping sounds slowed down. When they reached below the desired level, and his forehead was relaxed, the beeps turned off completely. Jonathan was fascinated to note that his muscle activity changed depending on the issues discussed. He realized that his body, not only his mind and his feelings, were responding to problem situations. This immediate audio feedback motivated Jonathan to learn more productive problem-solving skills to use at school, suggesting to us that not only his head would benefit!

Biofeedback teaches children that they can control aspects of their own behavior that they previously thought they could not influence. Thus, biofeedback increases children's autonomy and self-sufficiency.

Biofeedback requires specialized equipment and a trained health professional, both of which may be costly and can restrict its use. There are some simple feedback devices for ascertaining temperature, such as biobands, temperature-sensitive strips that are attached to a child's finger or forehead. These change color as the peripheral temperature changes, giving immediate feedback about the degree of success of focused concentration and relaxation and enabling the child to practice the self-regulation routine at home. Biobands can be helpful to children with migraine headaches who experience cold hands as an accompaniment to their headache. Research also suggests that routine relaxation training may be as effective as biofeedback in achieving relaxation, so it can be useful as a follow-up to biofeedback instruction.

MUSIC

Age: All ages
Pain: All types
Time: As long as desired

Music in its many forms—listening to a lullaby, singing, listening to an audio-tape, playing an instrument—can ease an atmosphere of suffering and tension. Music can be used as therapy to promote relaxation, harmony, and a sense of control, and can become a form of self-expression. Bringing a Walkman with a familiar tape into the treatment room during a painful routine spinal tap has provided an increased sense of control for numerous teenagers. Playing a favorite nursery rhyme on a tape recorder during a blood transfusion or other bothersome medical procedures has helped many toddlers and preschoolers get through the trying procedure in a comparatively pleasant way. Occasionally, a staff member bringing a guitar into the ward where a child is in pain has provided a much appreciated change.

Music is a wonderful way to bring the child's world harmoniously into the medical setting, supporting the well-being of the child and making long periods of time feel shorter, or at least more interesting. Singing along with a child, creating new verses, encouraging your child to create her own verses, or writing a song together as you travel to an appointment or are waiting at home can make time pass more pleasantly.

Music can be used as a form of therapy to foster self-expression or as encouragement during rehabilitation or a graduated physical exercise program. Music is easily transported from home to car to hospital, or to a park. It can be a fine aid in shifting attention away from pain and onto a very pleasant alternative. Music needs to be included more often in the treatment and recovery process for children. Parents sometimes worry that the child's music will be intrusive in the clinic or hospital. This is generally not the case; in fact, most staff members welcome the change of sounds.

PLAY AND ART

Age: 18 months and older
Pain: Pain that has upset the child, particularly treatment-related or persistent pain

Time: 10 to 45 minutes

Play is a natural part of every child's life. It is the child's way of understanding the world, of coming to terms with puzzling and complex occurrences, and of mitigating traumatic experiences. Play provides the child with an opportunity to assimilate these experiences into his growing sense of the world. Play therapy with a trained practitioner provides the child with a safe opportunity to express a range of emotions, thereby revealing the child's concept of the experiences.

Medical play provides young children with an opportunity to come to terms with the distressing experiences and separations of hospital life. Medical play or art therapy is of particular benefit for children undergoing recurring intensive treatments that involve multiple painful procedures, since these tend to undermine the child's psychological well-being. Trained child-life specialists, psychologists, and social workers can provide the following therapeutic opportunities for the child:

- Playing with a doctor's kit or with some of the medical equipment, such as putting a tourniquet on and off a non-favorite toy, to which the child is not emotionally attached.
- Using playdough to make figures that need or have experienced painful procedures and talking to them. This use of imagination allows the child to take on other roles, such as that of the nurse or doctor, and reveals the child's fantasy or concept of their motives and how the child perceives these people.
- Drawing; children's graphic drawings very powerfully reveal their inner world, their concerns, suffering, perceptions, and misunderstandings. With such visual information on hand, the issues are aired, providing some relief, and misconceptions can be corrected and clarified.
- Playing with puppets to help the child articulate more details of her experiences and to provide her with an opportunity to gain some control over distressing experiences.
- Keeping a journal that combines their drawings and with personal commentary recording the child's thoughts and feelings. Children can then look back to their journal to make sense of their experience at a later date. This method works well with older children.

In a safe context, using any or all of the items mentioned above, children will spontaneously express through play and talk, even within a hospital, what has been bottled up inside and is troubling them—information that may be helpful for the child's doctor or psychotherapist to know. Play is the child's natural medium of communication and is a means to recovery: being sick and in pain should not remove the child's right to have access to this source of pleasure and benefit.

CONTROL

Age: One year and older
Pain: Treatment-related, chronic, and acute pain
Time: As needed

Providing control for children in pain is more of a guiding principle than a distinct technique; there are, however, a number of behavioral methods that help give control to children in pain, such as using distraction and thought-stopping.

Feeling helpless is a natural consequence of being in pain or having to undergo painful procedures. Offering some control in situations that by custom don't lend themselves to it, such as having a painful procedure in a clinic or hospital, helps reduce feelings of helplessness and uncertainty. Having a few choices can change the meaning of the situation from "There's nothing that I can do that can make it different" to "Now that I have this control, I can get through this." There are a number of ways that children can be given areas of control:

Choosing how much information to receive. The amount of information a child wants is individual, varies from child to child, and is not related to the age or the sex of the child. Here are three children's comments from an interview study about how much information they would like to have about a medical intervention: A five-year-old boy said, "Don't tell me. I don't want to know nothing about it, okay?" In contrast a nine-year-old girl commented, "I like to know everything and how bad and I think about it a lot and then I'm ready, even if it's real bad, I'm ready." A twelve-year-old boy said: "The first time I go to a doctor or dentist for anything I get them to tell me all about it first. Then I check and find out if they're lying. It's best to know." Asking a child and knowing the child's temperament, coping style, and personal preferences helps in deciding how much information to give.

Being invited to make a genuine decision. For example, the child can be asked which arm to use for an injection or when to make a doctor's appointment.

Having partial control in the pacing of a procedure. For example, the child can decide how long to endure a procedure before calling for a halt (one child called it a hurting-break). By practicing self-pacing, the child knows he isn't helpless. This strategy is common in dental practice, when the child will put up a hand to indicate "stop" when a break is overdue. It is clear that choosing pauses increases the child's ability to tolerate and to endure the procedure.

Giving the child the choice about who will accompany her for the painful procedure or to the doctor's or dentist's. Children sometime choose a sibling, favorite relative, or grandparent.

Using an external control method suitable for young children. For example, pop-up books work well as a distraction strategy.

Using an inner control method. For example, thought-stopping (explained below) is ideal for school-aged children.

Distraction

Age: Ten months and older
Pain: Treatment-related, acute, and chronic pain
Time: As needed and usually for a short duration

Distraction is the active diverting of the child's attention—not tricking the child but inviting the child to shift attention onto a chosen interesting and more pleasant physical object than the painful procedure. The child can choose anything of interest, such as a special book, a musical toy, a magic wand, bubbles, or a colorful egg timer. The rationale is that since the pain experience depends on the processing of the pain information by the brain, distraction may interrupt or interfere with the processing of the sensory and emotional impulses in the brain. Distraction is most effective with mild pain, particularly pain that it is familiar to the child. The child will be more willing to shift attention away if the routine is known and holds no surprises.

- Bubbles can be a visual distractor. After the physical release of blowing the bubbles, the child can count the bubbles or track them until they pop.
- Focusing on objects in the room is an easy but short form of distraction, such as counting the flowers on Mom's blouse or tracking a musical toy as it completes its routine.
- Pop-up books provide multiple choices for diversion, surprise, and humor. The child has control over which tab to pull, can feel accomplishment when he can identify an object or number on the page, and can be delighted and surprised by the many and unexpected situations in these inventive books. (A list of the books most useful during painful procedures is included in Recommended Resources.)

The following case of the way three-year-old Meg and her mother managed a tough week in hospital illustrates how some of the methods discussed above can be creatively combined.

Meg had a rare eye cancer. In the course of treatment, she needed five consecutive days of IV therapy. Not surprisingly, by the third day she had learned what was in store for her and began kicking and crying when she was taken into the treatment room. Her mom, however, was prepared. She straddled the treatment table with Meg nestling between her legs and took out Meg's favorite book, "Curious George Goes to Hospital." She read the book in a loud, confident voice, asking Meg questions and making humorous remarks. Meg became involved in the story, but every now and again looked around the room. She tensed when the IV nurse entered the room and whimpered when the nurse began looking at the veins on her foot. Mom successfully distracted Meg's attention back to the book by saying: "Hey, what is Curious George doing on the telephone? Do you remember when Mommy accidentally phoned New York instead of Aunt Elsie?"

As the nurse began cleaning her foot, Meg's mom began blowing bubbles and then held the wand for Meg to blow. "Blow away the owies!" directed Mom firmly as Meg looked at the needle, blowing and whimpering. As the needle was inserted, her mom guided Meg's attention back to the story by saying, "Good, we'll soon have the Band-aid on. What on earth is Curious George up to now!" Her positive involvement, her physical containment of Meg, and her active direction of Meg's attention away from the source of pain to her loved story enabled Meg to finish the remaining days of that treatment with steadily diminishing anxiety and distress.

Thought-Stopping

Age: Six years and older
Pain: Anticipatory anxiety for medical and dental treatments
Time: Brief

A child can exert control in an internal way, such as using thought-stopping. Developed for children by Dr. Dorrie Ross, this method is particularly good for those who focus on and exaggerate the unpleasant aspects of the pain, called "catastrophizing." Thought-stopping teaches the child to catch himself as he begins to catastrophize and to deliberately substitute a positive thought. Children make up a positive statement, which they then memorize and repeat to themselves. Frederick, a seven-year-old boy on dialysis for his kidney condition, had an intense dislike of his dialysis machine:

"If I think about [the machine] I get real mad at myself, and I say 'Fred, you stop that thinking . . . STOP!' Then I say 'It's just two hours. My friends are here. The TV is on and I'll feel really good afterwards.' And if I start thinking about the machine again, I just say, 'Stop that thinking, you dumbbell, and say, 'It's just two hours' all over again and again!'"

The positive and reassuring aspects of the situation are condensed into key points. For example, for a feared blood draw, a child might say, "It'll be over quickly. I have good veins. The nurse who does it is nice." The child says this every time any negative thoughts pop back into her mind. Parents and staff can write the child's statement on a card until it is memorized. Children repeat their statement under their breath or aloud. With practice, the statements are reinforced and the previous fear and catastrophizing weakened. Thought-stopping provides a very easy first step in developing an independent coping strategy, a first step in controlling anxiety and developing skills that can then be extended to other methods.

All of the methods to relieve a child's pain that have been described in this chapter are effective and respectful ways of joining with a child or adolescent to manage and reduce pain. When used frequently, these methods develop into a coping repertoire for a child and help to forge strong bonds between child, parent, and pediatric staff.

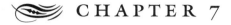 CHAPTER 7

Medication to Relieve Pain

Using Medication at Home

This section, written with Dr. Christy Scott, assistant professor at the School of Pharmacy at the University of North Carolina, provides information on over-the-counter and prescription pain medications that are available for use at home. It also provides some creative methods for encouraging children to take these sometimes difficult-to-swallow items, and tells you how long the various medications tend to be effective in reducing pain and what negative effects (or side effects) may occasionally occur.

A number of medications can be used at home to alleviate pain in children and adolescents. When you are talking to children about pain relief, "medication" is more useful than the term "drug." Because many people associate the use of drugs with street life and addiction, the word "drugs" has negative connotations. Parents and caregivers need to appreciate these connotations, since children in pain must be comfortable asking for and taking analgesic medication. They should know that medications taken for pain are a world apart from drugs taken for a "high" or as the result of psychological desperation and addiction.

SOME GUIDING PRINCIPLES

1. *For mild pain, such as toothache or mild headaches, give medication as soon as the pain is felt.* The sooner it is given, the faster the relief, preventing the buildup of pain and discomfort.

2. *For moderate to severe pain, such as that resulting from broken bones, sprained joints, surgery, or disease, give medication regularly, or "around the clock."* Pain relievers are given even if the pain is not felt in order to pre-

vent the pain from recurring. For example, if ibuprofen (a non-steroidal anti-inflammatory agent, see below) is used to treat pain from a sprained ankle, it should be given every six hours around the clock for about two to three days, or longer, if needed. (If a dose is given at 6:00 A.M., the next dose is due at 12 P.M., followed by another dose at 6.00 P.M. and another at 12:00 midnight—even if your child is not feeling pain at the time.) Providing medication around the clock usually requires waking a sleeping child, which is not easy to do, but it is essential if you want to ensure a pain-free and restful sleep. The child will awake with less pain and you will prevent the pain from occurring instead of treating the pain after it is felt.

Research has shown that less medication is required when pain medication is given to prevent pain, as opposed to giving medication to relieve pain. Therefore giving your child pain medication around the clock will keep your child comfortable and pain-free, allowing the child's energy to be used for healing and recovery instead of for dealing with pain.

3. *Ask how the medication needs to be administered.* It is your right to have directions properly and clearly explained. Your pharmacist and physician have a responsibility to ensure that you have all the information you require to give medication correctly to your child.

4. *Ask what effect the medication may have on your child.* Knowing the potential side effects is the best way to monitor the safety of the medication for your child.

5. *Read the label carefully, since some guidelines can be confusing.* If there are columns listing age, weight, and dosage, and your four-year-old falls into the weight category of the six- to seven-year-olds, follow the weight criterion. The child's body size determines how much medication is required.

6. *Give the full dose recommended for the age or weight of your child.* Using a lower dose will not provide the relief needed, and you will end up giving a more distressed child more medication to alleviate pain. The doses recommended at the different ages are safe and effective. Similarly, do not increase the recommended doses and times that the medication should be given. Even though many of these medications are over-the-counter products, they can cause severe problems if not administered properly. For example, if acetaminophen is given in excessive doses or too frequently, liver damage can occur.

7. *Combining medications may cause complications.* If your child is receiving other medications, ask your pharmacist or physician whether

the pain medications may be taken with them so that you can avoid any negative effects.

8. *Keep medications safely away from children.* Medication is often stored in the medicine cabinet in the bathroom. This is not the best place, since the heat and humidity may cause certain medications to break down more quickly. Children also know that medications are stored in the bathroom, increasing the risk of accidental overdoses. Medications should be kept in a cool, dry place away from children—for example, in the parents' bedroom, in a cabinet with a safety latch. Also, be sure to discard unused or outdated medications, since the more medications there are around, the greater the risk of confusion and accidental overdose.

9. *Choose and stay with one pharmacy.* Like choosing and staying with one physician, one hospital, and one dentist, choosing one pharmacy ensures that the pharmacists at that location will come to know you and your child and his or her condition and medications. With this available medication profile, the pharmacist can alert you to drug interactions and provide tips in administering, spacing, and assessing medications.

10. *When possible, choose generic rather than brand-name medications.* A number of prescription and over-the-counter pain medications have the same active ingredient (its generic name), although they are known by different names (their brand names, chosen by the manufacturers). The medications described in this chapter are listed alphabetically by their generic name, followed by common brand names in parentheses. Generic drug companies use some of the same active ingredients in medication that is usually available at a lower price than the brand names. Such products are known as generic products. Ask your pharmacist if a generic product is available for the medication you desire.

METHODS OF TAKING MEDICATIONS

Medications can be given to children by mouth, by rectum, or through the skin. Whatever the route, a parent or caregiver must discuss medications seriously with the child. The child needs an explanation of why the medication is being given, what it is intended to do, and how long it may take to work. The older the child, the more information you should convey. Be positive and firm. Do not let your anxieties about whether or not the child will take the medication cause you to lie or to mislead your child. For example, do not state that it doesn't taste bad when it does. Instead, discuss options and give your child choices. Let your child choose where and how to take the medication, what she would like to drink after it, and what reward she may have immediately afterward, such as eating a popsicle or hearing a story. You could say for example: "Susie, it is now time to take your medication, ibuprofen. Would you like to follow it with a glass of soda pop or a popsicle?" Or, "It is now time to take your medication, naproxen. Would you like to swallow it with a small amount of peanut butter or applesauce? While you're taking it, I can read the rest of the story to you."

By Mouth (Orally)

Generally, the best way for children to take medication is by mouth. Most medications are taken orally, in the form of tablets, capsules, and liquids. Generally, children under six are not able to easily swallow pills or capsules and manage liquids much better. These are usually sweetened or flavored to make them tolerable to swallow.

Liquids The best method for a child to swallow a liquid is to use an oral syringe, which is available at most pharmacies. The tip fits into the bottle of medication, allowing you to easily draw up the required dose. The syringe is clear, with markings to indicate the proper amount. Be careful not to squirt the medication back into the child's mouth, since this can cause the child to splutter, cough, or choke. Instead, slowly push the liquid into the side of the child's cheek so that it is easily swallowed. As children become familiar with the oral syringe, they sometimes prefer to give themselves the medication and do so with some pride.

Some children resist swallowing liquid medicine. Here are some considerations and alternative methods:

- Chilling the liquid medicine may weaken its taste, making it more tolerable. Immediately follow the "bad"-tasting medication with a carbonated drink, which helps to get the taste out of the child's mouth more quickly—and serves as a reward for taking the medication.
- If your child enjoys sucking ice, put ice on his tongue before and/or after he takes the medication, since it will numb the tongue. Similarly, allow your child to suck on a popsicle before and/or after giving the medication so that the treat becomes the highlight.

Do not mix medication in a bottle of milk or liquid. When medication is placed in a bottle, there is no way of ensuring that your baby or toddler will get the adequate dose. She may not finish the bottle, or it may take 15 or 20 minutes to finish the bottle, delaying and possibly reducing the effect of the medication. Instead, use an oral syringe and place it in the baby's or toddler's cheek, followed immediately by a bottle or breast to ensure that the medication is swallowed. Liquid chocolate can help hide a bitter taste.

- Liquid medications are more likely to taste bitter than tablets, since the liquid covers more surface area of the mouth and tongue than does the tablet. Mixing the medication with chocolate syrup can disguise the taste.

- After the child has taken the liquid, brush his teeth or have him brush his teeth. This is especially important with frequent, regular use of medication. A study has shown that children taking liquid medications chronically have an increased incidence of dental cavities because of the sugar content and acidity of most medications.

Pills Children aged six and older are usually able to swallow tablets and capsules. Capsules are usually easier to swallow because they are narrow and designed to shoot down the throat. Here are some tips and precautions:

- Teach the child to pop the tablet on the back of her tongue and swallow it while drinking a full glass of water. Usually after the second or third swallow the tablet will go down.

- Some children may find it easier to swallow the pill with a favorite cookie. Be sure, however, to follow up by giving your child a big drink to dissolve the analgesic tablet and promote its absorption.

- As long as the tablet isn't bitter or slow-release, crush the tablet finely and mix it in a half teaspoon of honey, which, as you know, helps the medicine go down!

- Bury the tablet in a teaspoon of jelly or ice cream, applesauce, peanut butter, or even a softened piece of chocolate. If the tablet is not labeled "extended" or "slow-release," it can be broken into a few pieces and similarly hidden in a small amount of food. A small amount (a teaspoon to a tablespoon) should be used to ensure that all of the food is eaten. Toddlers and preschool-aged children (aged one to four) generally put up the most resistance; therefore, crushing and hiding the medication in a small amount of food works best for this age group. Older children (aged five to eight) can more easily be reasoned with and involved in how best to take the tablet.

  A word of caution in using the child's favorite food. If your child resists taking medication and has to take this medication regularly, burying the medication in your child's favorite food may help on the first or second occasion. Because of its association with the medication, however, your child may learn within a short time to dislike that favorite food. For children with chronic pain, in particular, this must be avoided, since their favorite foods are a source of comfort. Jointly choosing an acceptable alternative food is preferable.

- Oral medications can cause stomach upset. Taking the medication with a small amount of food will ease the discomfort. In general, all *pain* medications can be taken with food. Other medications may require being taken on an empty stomach if they are not well absorbed when taken with food.
- With tablets and capsules, the child should drink a full glass of water, or another liquid, to ensure that the medication does not get stuck going down the throat; the liquid will also enhance the dissolving and absorption of the medication.
- Some medications come in "slow-release" or "extended-release" form. They need to be taken whole and not broken or chewed in order to maintain their longer activity, making them very difficult for younger children to take. Slow-release medications are not available in liquid form.

By rectum Medications that are administered by the rectum are understandably disliked by most children, who find them uncomfortable and embarrassing. Giving medication rectally should be reserved for children who are nauseated, or vomiting, or who refuse to or are unable to take their medications by swallowing. If it is unavoidable, be sure that your child understands the procedure and why you are giving the medication this way. One way of explaining it to a preschool-or school-aged child is as follows: "Your tummy is upset and has been throwing everything up. If you swallow your pain medication, it's not going to stay down and help your pain to go away. We want you to feel better and not be in this pain, so we need to use a suppository. It goes inside your bottom, and your body will absorb it and it will ease the pain. At first it will feel rather strange, and a little uncomfortable. This feeling will last a short time, and your bottom won't be sore."

Suppositories need to be stored in a cool, dry place, such as the refrigerator, to keep them firm. To put in a suppository, wash your hands and remove the foil wrapper. Moisten the suppository with *cool* water to help it enter the rectum easily. Have your child lie down on his side with the top leg bent. Talking all the time to your child and explaining what you are doing, use your finger to gently push the suppository up into the rectum until it disappears. (It does not have to be placed very high, just beyond the tight area of the rectum, the sphincter muscle.) If the suppository is too soft to insert, cool it in the refrigerator for 30 minutes before inserting it. Once it is in place, the child is free to move about.

Through the skin A few pain medications, primarily local anesthetics, are given through the skin (transdermally). Children tolerate and manage this application well. EMLA® (described in detail on the following pages) is a local anesthetic in cream or patch form, which is increasingly being used for pain associated with invasive procedures such as injections and placement of intravenous (IV) lines. It can be applied at home to prepare for clinical care. It also works indirectly on anxiety by removing the fear and anticipation of the pain. EMLA does not have any troublesome side effects.

Common pain medications for home use

The following are the pain medications that are available for use with children at home.

ACETAMINOPHEN
(Brand names: Tylenol®, Panadol®, Tempra®)
Available in liquids, tablets, capsules, and suppositories, acetaminophen is suitable for infants, young children, and children unable to take or keep food down.

Benefits
- Acetaminophen reduces fever and relieves pain due to toothaches, teething, ear infections, sore throats, mild menstrual pain, and some headaches.
- It is very well tolerated and considered safe in children.
- There is a great deal of experience with this medication in pediatric patients.
- Acetaminophen also causes very few side effects.

Drawbacks
- Acetaminophen has no anti-inflammatory properties, so if inflammation is causing the pain or adding to it, acetaminophen may

not be the most useful medication. Inflammation is present in muscle pain, sprained joints, toothaches, menstrual cramps, and cancer pain; therefore, for these pain conditions, other medications would probably be more useful, especially if it is not mild pain.

- If too much acetaminophen is taken, as in an overdose, it may lead to serious complications. Administer only the recommended amount, either with or without food or milk.

Use with codeine

For more severe pain in children, such as migraine headaches or some post-operative pain, acetaminophen combined with codeine may be useful. In Canada, acetaminophen with 8 mg codeine (Tylenol No. 1®) and acetaminophen with codeine elixir (Tylenol with codeine elixir®) are available without prescription. Acetaminophen with codeine in the amounts of 15, 30, and 60 mg (Tylenol No. 2®, 3®, and 4®, respectively) require a prescription because of the higher codeine content. In the United States, all acetaminophen with codeine formulations, some of which contain slightly different amounts of codeine from the Canadian products, require a prescription.

ASPIRIN/ACETYLSALICYLIC ACID
(*Brand names: Bayer®, Ecotrin®, and many more*)

Aspirin is available in tablets, chewable tablets, and suppositories. A liquid product is not available.

Circumstances under which aspirin may be used

- Inflammation in the heart following heart surgery
- Juvenile rheumatoid arthritis

Aspirin has long been used and found to be helpful in these conditions of inflammation in adults and children, since its benefits outweigh its risks.

Precautions

- Aspirin should only be used by those who are over 16 years old. In very special circumstances and under direct physician supervision, it may be used by children under 16. When taken by children, aspirin can cause Reye's syndrome, resulting in liver and brain damage and possibly coma and death. Reye's syndrome has been associated with children who have had a fever with the flu or other viral illnesses and taken aspirin at the same time. If your child is receiving aspirin and develops a fever, the flu, or chicken pox, it may be best to stop administering the medication. Discuss the signs of a viral infection with your physician or pharmacist.

- Because aspirin may provoke an asthmatic attack in children and teenagers with asthma, they should avoid taking this medication.
- Aspirin decreases some clotting activity in the blood and therefore can cause bleeding problems if taken regularly. If your child is going for surgery, aspirin use should be stopped five to seven days before surgery. If dark, tarry stools are noted, stop administering the medication immediately. This may mean internal bleeding has occurred, and your child's physician or pharmacist should be notified.

Side Effects

Aspirin may cause stomach upset. It is advisable to administer aspirin with food or milk to decrease irritation to the stomach. A full meal is acceptable but not necessary; a few crackers, spoonfuls of applesauce or cottage cheese, or other small amounts of food are all that is needed. It is also best to take aspirin with a full glass of water (6 to 8 ounces). Your child should not lie down afterward because it can cause a burning feeling in the esophagus. Some brands of aspirin have a protective coating to decrease distress to the stomach. This type of product does not need to be taken with food, but it must be swallowed whole to keep its protective covering intact; therefore, children under six may have a difficult time swallowing it.

IBUPROFEN
(*Brand names: Advil®, Medipren®*)

Ibuprofen is a pain reliever with anti-inflammatory properties similar to those of aspirin. Reye's syndrome, however, does not appear to be a problem with this medication.

Available in non-prescription strength in Canada, ibuprofen comes only in tablet form, thus making it difficult to use with children under six years of age, when most children learn to swallow tablets. Ibuprofen is under "pharmacist control" in Canada and is kept behind the pharmacy counter. It is necessary to ask the pharmacist for ibuprofen and state why you wish to use the medication. Ibuprofen is also available in prescription strength. In the United States, ibuprofen is readily available over the counter, wherever aspirin and acetaminophen are sold, and also comes in liquid form (PediProfen®), which has recently become available without a prescription.

What it is used for

Ibuprofen is effective for pain associated with inflammation, including pain from juvenile rheumatoid arthritis, sprained joints, broken bones, headaches, and menstrual pain. Ibuprofen, like acetaminophen and aspirin in older children, may also be used to treat fever.

Side effects

- This medication may cause stomach upset. It is best to administer ibuprofen with food or milk to decrease any irritation to the stomach. A full meal is acceptable but not necessary; a few crackers or spoonfuls of applesauce or cottage cheese or other small amounts of food are all that is needed. It is also best for your child to take a full glass of water (6 to 8 ounces) with this medication and not to lie down for 15 minutes afterwards, decreasing any potential for stomach upset.
- Ibuprofen has the rare potential to cause bleeding problems, much like aspirin. If your child is going for surgery, it is important to stop administering ibuprofen two days before surgery. If dark, tarry stools are noted while your child is taking ibuprofen, stop administering the medication. This may mean internal bleeding is occurring, and your child's physician or pharmacist should be notified.

Similar medications

There are many other medications within the same class as ibuprofen, known as nonsteroidal anti-inflammatory drugs (or NSAIDs). These include naproxen, diclofenac, indomethacin, and tolmetin, among many others. Naproxen is now available over the counter, but only for adults. All of the other medications require a prescription. Naproxen is the only other product (besides ibuprofen, in the U.S.) available in liquid form, both in Canada and the United States.

PRILOCAINE AND LIDOCAINE CREAM
(*Brand name:* EMLA®)

EMLA® is a white cream that was recently developed to provide numbness (local anesthesia) in small areas of intact skin. It consists of two local anesthetics, prilocaine and lidocaine, that have been blended together into a cream base, which can be directly applied to the skin in the area where a puncture will occur. Note that it only works where it is applied.

In Canada, EMLA® is available without a prescription, but it should not be used for infants under six months without advice from a physician. In the United States a prescription is required, but EMLA® is available for use with infants one month and older.

What it is used for

EMLA® is used to minimize pain during the following procedures:

- When a needle enters into the skin, as in needle sticks for blood drawing, IV starts, immunization shots, dialysis, and lumbar punctures
- For superficial surgical procedures, such as the removal of small warts
- Laser treatment for the removal of port wine stains.

EMLA® is a helpful and effective medication for children who must undergo many painful procedures because of their illness, since it has a wide safety margin.

How it is used

- To be effective, EMLA® must be applied to the skin for a *minimum* of 60 minutes to a maximum of four hours and longer for darker skin. For minor procedures, leave the cream in place for at least one hour and two hours for deeper procedures, such as mole or wart removal. When the cream is removed, anesthesia will continue to increase for another 15 minutes, since there is a reservoir of anesthetic built up in the skin.

  After a 60-minute application time, the cream will penetrate 3 mm into the skin, and this depth will increase to 5 mm two hours after application. Therefore, the procedure does not have to occur immediately. After two hours, however, the cream will not penetrate any further into the skin and the anesthesia will gradually begin to wear off. The loss of anesthesia usually occurs within two hours but may take up to five hours, depending on many factors, such as how much blood is delivered to that tissue.

- When the medication is wiped off, the area usually looks slightly blanched and will be numb. Your child should not feel the pain associated with the procedure, even though she will know the procedure is being done and there may be some stinging during an immunization. It thus remains important to talk to and comfort your child, since the procedure may still be a scary experience.

Precautions

Currently EMLA® is not indicated for use near the middle ear, or the eye, or on burns or open wounds. If used on wounded skin, some of the medication may be absorbed and your child may be at risk for systemic side effects, such as problems involving the blood. A by-product of the local anesthetic is that it causes vasoconstriction at low doses and vasodilation at higher doses, so you may see mild whitening or mild reddening of the skin.

Availability

EMLA® is available in a tube (5 and 30 grams) with or without a special bandage, or you can obtain an all-in-one patch in which the cream is already embedded in the patch. If you use the tube form, apply a thick layer of EMLA® to the area where local anesthesia is needed, generally an area the size of a loonie or a silver dollar. Depending on his or her size, a child will usually require half of a 5-gram tube. Place the special bandage that comes with the packaging over the designated area and seal the bandage tightly. This bandage, known as an occlusive dressing, helps the medication to work by increasing the contact EMLA® has with the skin. Note that EMLA® will not work if it is not occluded with the enclosed bandage.

DOSES AND EFFECTS OF MEDICATION

Table 8.3 provides a brief summary of important information about medications that may be used for treating pain at home, including dosing directions. To determine the dose of the particular medication, multiply the child's weight in kilograms by the dose in milligrams in the table. If you know your child's weight in pounds, divide the number by 2.2 to convert the weight into kilograms. For example, if your child weighs 20 pounds, this is equal to about 10 kilograms. If you need to give acetaminophen, the dose is 10 milligrams per kilogram. Therefore, the dose would be 100 milligrams. If you are using a liquid preparation, ask your pharmacist for an oral syringe to measure the dose properly.

Medications Used in Hospital for Pain Relief

A child who is in hospital may experience more severe pain and require more potent pain medication to obtain relief than at home. The following section describes some of the most common analgesic medications, such as opioid analgesics, and their delivery through patient-controlled analgesia (PCA), which may be used for your child during a hospital stay. Some of these medications may also be prescribed by your child's physician for continued use at home.

NONSTEROIDAL ANTI-INFLAMMATORY DRUGS (NSAIDS)

There are many medications within this category, including ibuprofen (Motrin®, Advil®), naproxen (Naprosyn®), tolmetin (Tolectin®), and sulindac (Clinoril®). These medications decrease inflammation and provide pain relief. They may be prescribed for children with juvenile rheumatoid arthritis either in hospital or at home. Children with bone pain from cancer may receive one of these medications along with an opioid medication, such as morphine, for added effect. Since inflammation is associated with bone pain, anti-inflammatory medications decrease this pain, and in conjunction with an opioid, many children find satisfactory relief for this very painful condition. (Please see Ibuprofen under Medications at Home, above, for a more detailed explanation of these medications.)

OPIOID ANALGESICS

The opioid medications, also known as narcotics, are very potent and effective pain relievers and include the following medications: codeine, morphine, meperidine (Demerol®), hydromorphone (Dilaudid®), and fentanyl. Morphine is commonly used in hospital because it has been studied the most in children and health care professionals are most comfortable with its use. Opioid analgesics are frequently used for children following surgery, or with cancer pain, and sometimes in the intensive care unit for children who require continuous pain relief and sedation because of painful procedures and extra "instrumentation" (such as intravenous lines, a ventilation tube, chest tubes).

Concerns about addiction

Some parents may worry that their child will become addicted to opioids medication. But this fear is based on a misunderstanding. When these medications are used appropriately for the treatment of pain, they are very effective and safe; they should not be confused with street drug use. Addiction from opioids occurs when people desire the "high" feeling that these medications can provide. Children (and adults) who need these medications for pain control are not seeking a "high" feeling; they are seeking relief from their pain. When they are used appropriately, opioids provide effective pain relief and addiction is not a concern.

Children (and adults) may become physically dependent on these medications, however. Physical dependence is very different from addiction. If a child has received opioid analgesics for longer than seven to ten days, the child's body becomes accustomed to having opioids and requires the medication to prevent physical withdrawal symptoms. Symptoms of withdrawal include feeling very uncomfortable, feeling restless, feeling achy, sweating, yawning, and having diarrhea. These symptoms can be easily controlled by slowly weaning the child off the medication, and the child will not have any psychological symptoms of withdrawal.

Methods of administering opioids

These medications can be given by different routes, including by mouth, by intramuscular injection, by intravenous injection or infusion, or into the spinal column (epidurally).

By mouth Usually, while your child is in hospital, the oral route is not used at first because of nausea, sleepiness, or discomfort. If necessary, however, your child may be sent home on oral medication. The liquid preparation may be given with a glass of juice to disguise its poor taste. If your child is receiving a long-acting preparation, such as MS Contin®, the tablet must be swallowed whole. It must not be crushed or halved, since too much medication would be released at once, leading to overdose, and it would lose its longer activity.

By intramuscular injection Opioid analgesics can be given by intramuscular injections (IM), which are very painful, are feared by most children, and therefore should be avoided. Many physicians still prescribe analgesics by the IM route, given as an injection every two to four hours, depending on which agent is used. If your child has a IV line in place, or requires a number of medications during the day and evening and therefore would do well to have an IV put in place, be sure to suggest the IV route to the staff. After the initial pain of accessing the vein, the intravenous route is not painful and provides quicker relief and a steady control of pain.

By intravenous line The IV infusion affords the best relief by providing a constant level of medication in the child's body while the pain lasts. Occasionally while the child is receiving a continuous infusion, another injection of the medication is required for painful procedures or when your child is feeling a lot of pain or is especially uncomfortable. This extra dose is called a bolus. The dose can easily be put directly into the intravenous line without another painful needle.

Spinal Opioid Infusion Opiod medication, usually morphine or fentanyl, may be infused by catheter into a small space in the spine known as the epidural space. This method is usually reserved for severe pain, such as after major surgery. The advantages of this route of administration are that smaller doses of medication are required, and the child is not as sleepy. Because of the catheter placement, however, the child may not be as mobile as when receiving medications intravenously. A side effect that may occur that does not usually appear with other routes of opioid administration is itching of the child's arms, trunk, and nose. Any side effects are manageable with proper nursing care, making spinal or epidural infusions a safe and effective method for pain management.

Patient-Controlled Analgesia (PCA) Using Patient-Controlled Analgesia, the child administers the opioid medication when she feels pain. By pressing a button located at the bedside (which is attached to a medication pump), a prepared amount of opioid will be infused though an intravenous line to the child. Through PCA, the child is in complete control of her own analgesic needs. For many reasons PCA is a useful method for the administration of opioids. Following are some of its advantages.

- Consistent blood levels of the analgesic can be maintained, usually by steadily administrating a "background opioid infusion." The background infusion supplies a low level of constant opioid infusion, and the child then administers the extra (bolus) doses as she requires, such as for dressing changes or physical therapy, or if she wakes up and feels in pain.
- PCA allows for adequate pain control without excessive sedation, because the child is in charge of how much medication is administered. Studies have demonstrated that patients require less medication for pain control using PCA than other methods.
- PCA has wide acceptance by physicians, pharmacists, nurses, parents, and, most important, children. There are usually age limits on the use of PCA. Most hospitals that offer PCA to children require that the child be at least ten years old and understand the purpose and operation of PCA.

Other hospitals may offer the service to younger children, such as seven-year-olds, if they are deemed capable. Some hospitals also allow "Parent-Controlled Analgesia" or "Nurse-Controlled Analgesia," where either the parent or the nurse administers the medication through the same method as PCA for a young child in chronic pain. We encourage you to ask if any of these services are available for your child in acute pain.

Side Effects of Opioids

All of the opioid analgesics tend to cause the same side effects. The side effects of these medications may appear extensive at first, but almost all may be controlled.

- Your child will probably be sleepy, especially for the first one to three days. This effect, as well as changes in behavior and mood, usually resolves within the first day or two of treatment. Expect these changes, but realize they will not last forever.
- Your child's pupils may become pinpoints. This is an effect the medication has on the pupil itself and is not a problem, since it does not affect your child's vision. Opioid medications may also cause your child's mouth to become dry. Your child may suck on ice chips, popsicles, or candies to relieve the dryness.
- One of the most often cited concerns when a child is given opioid medications is that of "respiratory depression," which occurs infrequently, especially when the medication is administered in the proper doses. If too much morphine is given, children can have problems breathing. If respiratory depression does occur, however, your child may receive naloxone, a medication that works very quickly to reverse the effects of morphine and relieve any respiratory depression. With appropriate use of opioid medication, respiratory depression should not be a concern.
- Your child may become nauseated or vomit when taking one of the opioid medications. If your child is able to communicate with you, you should ask your child how his tummy is feeling. There are other medications that can be used to help relieve this problem. Sometimes these symptoms may be related to the slowing down of digestion, so being upright or lying on the right side may help.
- Constipation is a common problem with opioid medications and is usually evident after about two to three days of treatment. If possible,

make sure that your child receives plenty of fluids and request that stool softeners be prescribed with the medication to prevent constipation or to treat it.

- Sometimes your child may not be able to urinate effectively; this condition is known as urinary retention. Reminding your child to urinate can be helpful, but some children may require the short-term use of a catheter.

- Itching can also occur with these medications and is most common when they are given epidurally. Very small doses of naloxone may be given along with the medication to relieve this problem without reversing the pain-relieving effects.

Continuing morphine use at home

Morphine is also available in a liquid form for use at home, as well as in a slow-release tablet form (MS Contin®) for children older than six, if they are still experiencing persistent severe pain when they are discharged from hospital. Frequently a stool softener or laxative is also prescribed to prevent constipation. For the reasons already discussed, if your child is prescribed these medications for use at home, do not abruptly discontinue their use if he or she has received them for longer than one or two weeks. A slow decrease in the medication over five days to two weeks is best, depending on how long the child has received them. Your pharmacist can help you design a weaning schedule that is most appropriate for your child.

Hospitals are not perfect places, and omissions and mistakes can happen. Parents do not need to be anxious watchdogs, but they do need to know that they have a right to track their child's pain medications to ensure that their child's pain is well controlled.

PART III

How to Provide Relief in Different Situations

CHAPTER 8

Managing Pain At Home

Miss Molly had a baby, she named him "Tiny Tim"
She put him in the bathtub to see if he could swim
He drank a bottle of water, he ate a bar of soap,
He tried to eat the bathtub, but it wouldn't go down his throat.
Miss Molly called the doctor, the doctor called the nurse,
Miss Molly called the lady with the alligator purse.
In came the doctor, in came the nurse,
In came the lady with the alligator purse.
"Measles" said the doctor, "a shot" said the nurse,
"Pizza" said the lady with the alligator purse.
Out walked the doctor, out walked the nurse
Out walked the lady with the alligator purse.

CHILDREN UNDERSTAND THAT MISHAPS OCCUR at home, and as the chant reveals, they also have a concept of how to manage the pain from these mishaps that is beginning to approximate an adult's understanding. Unlike toddlers, school-aged children regard hurts at home not as a punishing or bewildering experience but often as something that can be diagnosed and treated.

"Why do I have so many owies, Mommy?" asked Rayush, aged three. A child's natural curiosity often leads to startled hurts and surprise injuries. Apart from incidental minor pain, it has been estimated that approximately 15 percent of children at some point have to manage pain as part of their lives, either as recurring pain or as chronic pain from a disease, serious trauma, or rehabilitation. The suggestions for managing acute pain, however, must not supplant consulting a good first-aid manual (see Recommended Resources) or your child's physician. Manuals

frequently neglect the emotional and interpersonal aspects of successfully coping with the pain situation and do not lay the groundwork for
using the situation to cope with future pain.

When a Child Has Acute Pain at Home

"Pain is what hurts," said a cogent six-year-old, holding his fractured
arm. Injuries are the source of the most serious form of pain commonly
experienced by children, and home is where injuries frequently occur:
cuts, bruises, broken bones, burns, lacerations, and other injuries are
the most common. Hurts like these often happen in the kitchen, where
there is a profusion of dangerous implements, and while playing, fighting with a sibling, or simply running around. Parents, babysitters, and
other caregivers all need to respond quickly and appropriately, to assess
the injury, and to make a decision whether or not the injury can be dealt
with at home without seeking immediate professional attention. If you
are unsure, remember that the emergency department of your nearest
hospital is only a phone call away. Keep a list of emergency phone numbers next to your telephone. These should include numbers for the local
emergency department, your pediatrician, the ambulance, the fire, and
local poison control center, and a trusted neighbor.

If you decide to call the nurse on duty or your child's physician, it is
helpful to provide the following information:

- Describe the nature of the injury and how it looks.
- Briefly describe what happened.
- Describe the child's response, what the child says about the injury and
  pain.
- Request help in deciding whether this acute pain can be treated at
  home or whether it requires prompt medical attention.

BABYSITTERS

It is vital that you tell your babysitters what should be done about accidents and injuries. Babysitters, like parents, often feel guilty when a child
is hurt. Some may even attempt to hide the injury from the child's parents. Thus, in the beginning of your relationship with your babysitter:

- Talk openly about the possibility that accidents can happen.
- Take the time to show the babysitter where the emergency phone
  numbers are.*

* In the United States, depending on the state, doctors may be legally unable to

- Tell him or her who can be called (including a trusted friend).
- Show the babysitter where your medications for cut and scrapes and the first-aid manual are stored.
- Go over the key contents of your medication cabinet and discuss how to treat minor hurts and major incidents.
- Write out a brief plan of your discussed action and leave it in an easily accessible place, perhaps with the emergency phone numbers.
- Stress that you value an open relationship and that in entrusting your child to the babysitter's care, you want to be kept informed about all important occurrences and accidents. (Parents leaving children who experience recurring or chronic pain have different concerns, which are covered later in this chapter.)

TREATMENT OF ACUTE PAIN AT HOME

Table 9.1 provides examples of relief for common minor and not-so-minor hurts that happen fairly frequently at home. By addressing not only the medical needs but also the fears and psychological needs as the pain occurs here, you can help your child develop a less fearful attitude toward his or her body and subsequent pain.

Table 8.1 Providing Relief For Acute Pain At Home

Minor Pain	Relief
Bleeding	The sight of blood is startling and frightening for children and may prompt crying even if the child isn't in pain. Immediately address this fear, whatever else is happening; normalize the presence of the blood by noticing its beautiful red color, or how healthy it looks, while you reach for a sterile gauze. While you apply direct and firm pressure on the wound and maintain it with the sterile gauze, describe to the child how his blood is doing an excellent job of cleaning the wound and how soon, very soon, it will stop bleeding. The bleeding should

provide routine emergency medical care for children aged either 14 or 16 years and younger without a parent release form. They will provide treatment only in life-threatening situations. It is therefore recommended that you have on hand a dated standard medical release form signed by the custodial parent and stating the child's name that authorizes a physician and hospital to provide necessary medical treatment. A form developed in cooperation with the American College of Emergency Physicians is available from McNeil Consumer Products (see Recommended Resources for the address).

Minor Pain	Relief
	stop within 15 minutes; if not, get immediate medical attention.
Cut finger, arm, leg	Place the wounded area under cool running water for up to five minutes, focusing the child's attention on the coolness and flow of water. The running water removes debris, cleans the wound, and cools the burning sensation. Absorb your child in the comforting sound and the familiar sight of the running water. Your child can sit at the kitchen sink or in a bathtub and use the taps or a hand-held shower. Explain to your child that cleaning the cut thoroughly prevents any foreign matter from lodging in the wound and starting an infection; it also soothes the hurting nerves and the skin. (Note that cuts longer than 1/2 inch or 1/4 inch on the child's face may need sutures.)
Bruises	Apply ice wrapped in a towel, a cold compress, or one of the frozen sponges described on p. 126 to the bruised area and hold it there for 10 to 15 minutes to provide comfort. Encourage your child to focus on the cool, soothing sensation of the ice as it penetrates the bruise and helps it to heal. Do not massage or give aspirin, since these actions may increase the bleeding (see chapter 7, under Aspirin). If further pain relief is needed, give acetaminophen. Tell your child that she will be able to notice the bruise healing because the bruise will change color from red to blue, then to yellow, and then possibly to brown—some bruises even have a greenish tinge— all interesting signs of healing that can be tracked.
Scrapes	Clean scrapes or abrasions thoroughly to help prevent infections. Since removing debris from a wound is very painful, it is important that your child use some self-regulation method, such as breathing, blowing bubbles, counting, squeezing a hand, or using active imagery while the wound is thoroughly washed under running water and the foreign matter gently removed. Whatever effort the child is putting forth needs to be actively supported and encouraged. Allow the child recovery time during the process, since it can be very painful. Let the abrasion dry exposed to the air, unless it is on the

Minor Pain	Relief
	child's feet or hands and is likely to get dirty; then apply a sterile non-stick dressing or a "magic" Band-aid.

Table 8.2

Not So Minor Pain	Home Intervention /Relief
Scalding and thermal burns	Immediately run cold water over the burn, continuing for ten minutes or longer until the pain stops. Tell the child to concentrate on the coldness of the water and to absorb all of its coldness. The application of cold lessens the depth of the burn and may promptly relieve the acute pain. You can coach your child with images of playing in the snow or of other cold activities. If there are blisters, leave them intact and have them assessed medically. Do not use butter or any ointments, since they keep the heat in. Give the child acetaminophen at the recommended dosage. If you are on the way to getting medical attention, keep the burned area in cold water or wrapped with frozen peas or crushed ice in a towel to lessen the pain.

Note: Deeper burns, known as third-degree burns, are burns in which all layers of the skin have been burned and open flesh is visible. Often the wound is painless, for in that area all the nerves have been destroyed, although the surrounding area may be very painful and your child may be in shock. In this situation do not apply cold water. Keep the child warm and feeling safe by covering him with a clean sheet and blanket, and call for immediate medical help or an ambulance.

Sunburn	After the sun has done its damage, there is a two- to four-hour delay in the appearance of symptoms. Pain, redness, and swelling may take 24 hours or more to appear, whereas a fever may appear in 12 to 24 hours. The skin of infants is thinner and very sensitive to the sun. The sun's rays are most intense, and therefore the most dangerous, between 10:00 a.m. and 2:00 p.m. Sunburn is both painful and potentially dangerous because it puts your child at risk of skin cancer later in life.
	If you suspect your child has a sunburn, immediately move her into the shade and give her a cool drink while you explain what has happened and

Not So Minor Pain	*Home Intervention /Relief*

how important it is that she be cooled down. While you examine the area, remember that it will take a few more hours for the full damage to be visible. Minor sunburn, which turns the skin pink or red, is a first-degree burn. Blistering, caused by prolonged exposure to the sun, is a sign of second-degree burn.

To relieve pain and discomfort, let your child soak in a cool bath with a couple of tablespoons of baking soda, or apply a cool compress (cloth or sponge) to the painful area. Avoid showers, since they can irritate the skin more. Drinking extra water helps to prevent dizziness and dehydration.

Note: The pain sensation can last for 48 hours. You can make your child more comfortable with acetaminophen or ibuprofen, given as soon as possible and continued for 12 to 24 hours to reduce inflammation and pain. Do not give aspirin in the presence of a fever. Consult your doctor if your child appears sick or is dizzy, if your child's temperature is 102°F (39°C) or over, or if the sunburn is blistering, widespread, and painful.

Dislocations or Fractures	If the injured part is deformed, swollen, or very painful, it may be fractured. Tell the child to stay very still until you splint and provide support for the bones to prevent further damage, and explain as calmly as you can what you are doing: "You're doing well, staying so still while I wrap your arm to give the sore part support so that it can feel more comfortable." Use your first-aid manual for splinting directions and call for the necessary help. If you are unsure whether or not a back or neck injury has occurred, do not move your child at all until emergency medical help arrives.

Your child may start shivering; this is a physical shock reaction and not necessarily fear. Talk soothingly, wrap the child with a warm blanket, and explain where you are going and why. Remind your child that his body knows how to heal as you take him for immediate medical care.

Abdominal pain	Abdominal pain (see also p. 186) must be first assessed by the child's physician. Since many different organic diseases can cause pain in the stomach, a careful and thorough medical examination is always the first step. A detailed history of the pain, pro-

Not So Minor Pain	Home Intervention /Relief
	vided by child and parents, is a great help in identifying possible causes. Abdominal pain in a child under two years of age and in a child whose tummy is very tender to touch or is bloated and hard needs immediate medical attention. If your child looks ill, is in severe pain, or is vomiting or feverish, the pain is a signal that something serious may be happening internally. Abdominal pain can be caused by an acute urinary tract infection, appendicitis, bowel disease, or an inflammatory bowel syndrome, among other causes.
	Commonly, however, children will not be diagnosed with a specific illness. Ten to 15 percent of school-aged children have abdominal pains that recur, and less than 10 percent in that group have any organic disease. If the pain is mild and not sharply acute, relieve it with a hot water bottle, a warm bath, a gentle tummy massage, and rest, and, for a young child, a good cuddle while you read a book together or listen to music. Children of elementary school age tend to have the highest incidence of abdominal pain, and kindergarten is a peak period for Monday morning stomach aches.
	Emotions exert a decisive influence on the body, and the soft abdomen is a key vulnerable site for children. Take the time to explore with your child what else besides the pain has been bothering, upsetting, or frightening her. Sometimes it can take a while for a child or teen to find the words or the confidence to put it all together. Allow for the necessary "breathing room" in your talk for that to occur

When a Child Has Chronic or Recurring Pain

Life changes in a multitude of ways for parents when a child's pain doesn't go away, but recurs or becomes chronic, embedding itself in the child's life. This pain can be associated with a chronic disease, such as cancer, arthritis, sickle cell disease, or AIDS, or the pain can be the problem itself, as with recurrent or chronic headaches, abdominal pains, menstrual cramps (dysmenorrhea), or limb pains that are not disease related and are known as "growing pains."

Table 8.3 Doses and Effects of Medication

Medication	Form	Dose given each time	Frequency	Onset of Action	Peak effect	Side effects and what to do
acetaminophen	liquid, tablet, capsule, suppository	10–15 milligrams per kilogram up to 650 milligrams	every four to six hours	within 30 minutes	one hour	rash rarely—stop medication; use only in recommended doses
aspirin	tablets, suppository	10–15 milligrams per kilogram up to 650 milligrams; much higher doses (i.e. 25 mg/kg per dose) may be needed for arthritic conditions	every four to six hours	within 30 minutes	one hour	do not use in children under 16 years unless under the care of a physician; stomach upset: take with food; bleeding: stop medication
ibuprofen	tablet	5–10 milligrams per kilogram up to 400 milligrams	every six hours	within 30 minutes	one hour	stomach upset: take with food; bleeding: stop medication
EMLA	cream for topical use	thick coating at site where injection is to be given	only one application is necessary	60–90 minutes for minor procedures, 2–3 hours for major procedures	60 minutes lasting 3–5 hours, after cream is removed	rarely, a rash in the area of application; do not apply again

Recurrent and chronic pains afflict children who are otherwise healthy. The conditions may not be life-threatening, but they can be difficult to live with, especially when the pain is not the symptom of an underlying disease but is the disorder itself. The episodes of pain can vary greatly in length, frequency, and intensity. They can be brought on or exacerbated by internal and external stress factors—for example, when parents are arguing, separating, or divorcing, a family member has died, the family is moving, or there are changes and pressures at school.

Adjusting to life with chronic pain can be protracted and exceedingly challenging, depending on whether a disease or trauma is involved or the pain itself persists with no end in sight. With recurring pain, the unpredictability of the pain episodes, as well as the uncertainty of the pain relief, can make children, parents, and families feel helpless. With chronic pain, the parents and child can feel worn down by the continual episodes of pain and may lose faith in their health care providers, believing that effective pain control and relief may no longer be possible.

The sooner the child and parents develop a repertoire of coping and pain-relieving skills with the regular support of a qualified clinician, the better off they will be. It is crucial to the long-term management of both recurring and disease-related persistent pain that parents actively search for health practitioners who

- recognize their child's pain and its impact on their child and family;
- make a long-term commitment to develop an effective course of treatment, which often involves a combination of changes in life-style, medication, physical therapies, and other self-regulatory methods; and
- encourage and enhance the coping skills of both parent and child so that as a team they can become knowledgeable participants in dealing with the pain.

MANAGING RECURRING PAIN AT HOME

The four most common recurring childhood pains managed at home are recurring abdominal pain, headaches, menstrual cramps (dysmenorrhea), and limb pains.

Recurring Abdominal Pain

Possible causes Recurring stomach or abdominal pain that is not disease related is very common in childhood and may be caused by constipation, indigestion, or internal or interpersonal stress. Clinical studies indicate that a multitude of factors may play a role in recurring abdominal pains:

the function of the entire gut, genetic disposition, family behavior, stress, a sensitive temperament, and the reactivity of the child's autonomic nervous system. For many children, the abdomen is a sensitive center of emotion; those who do not work out their distress through talking or "playing it out" do so in the physical expression of pain (a "worry" stomach or bowel). This does not mean that the child's abdominal pain is "all in his head"; the pain in his abdomen is real and distressing. As discussed earlier, our bodies are not divided along mental and physical lines. Our body systems are tightly interconnected and continually interact. Emotional distress nearly always has a physical expression, and physical pain nearly always has an emotional counterpart.

Controlling the pain A closer understanding of and support for the child's concerns, together with an improved diet and better pain management methods, can relieve abdominal pain. More specifically:

- If your child's bowel movements are not regular, a high-fiber diet of increased grains, especially bran, fruit, and vegetables, is one of the best steps you can take to help your child's bowels movements to become regular. A high-fiber diet (*Childhood Constipation and Soiling*, listed in Recommended Resources, explains how the bowel works and provides bran recipes) can maintain your child's regularity and reduce bowel pain, gas, and cramps. Keep in mind, however, that when you start a high-fiber diet the gas and pain may briefly increase before improvement follows.
- The help of a child psychotherapist, skilled in understanding the connections between mind, emotions, and body, can help the child and family to work through and to resolve whatever tensions have contributed to the child's pain and distress.

Headaches

Recurrent headaches can be caused by many combinations of emotional and physiological stress—for example, irregular eating habits; poor sleep; sinus congestion; muscle tension in the back, neck, and head; teenage girls' monthly hormonal changes; genetic inheritance; and stress, including difficulties with school, peers, and family. Such headaches warrant a full medical examination so that an infection, disease, or other concerns can be ruled out.

Headaches tend to be categorized into two groups, migraine headaches and tension headaches, although they can overlap, particularly when the headaches are more severe. Other, less common forms, such as sinus headaches, associated with congested sinuses, and cluster headaches, occur mostly in adults and only rarely in children or adolescents.

Migraine headaches These are predominantly vascular, resulting from changes in blood flow through the vessels in the brain. Contributing factors may include muscle tension, food sensitivities, and stress. Pain from migraine headaches is severe and throbbing and often occurs on one side of the head but may move from side to side. The pain is sometimes accompanied by nausea or vomiting. Sometimes the child may experience disturbances in her body sensation or visual field (known as an "aura") or may become very sensitive to light or noise. The pain can be severe: a seven-year-old boy described his migraine pain to two researchers, Drs. Dorothy and Sheila Ross, as follows: "Like there's this big monster in there, see, and he's growing like crazy and there's no room and he's pulling the two sides of my head apart he's getting so big."

It is incorrect to assume that very young children do not experience migraines. Children who are diagnosed with migraine at age seven or eight can sometimes trace this pain back to their early childhood years. Over 70 percent of children and teenagers with migraine headaches have close family members with similar headaches, underlining the strong genetic influence in their occurrence. The genetic influence, however, is a predisposition for developing migraines; stress triggers are then needed to bring on a migraine episode.

Incidence of migraines
- Before adolescence the incidence for girls and boys is equal.
- Migraines most commonly begin in the early teenage years, when girls tend to have a higher incidence rate than do boys.
- Hormonal factors play a role in the frequency of migraines, and it is known that contraceptive pills can also trigger the onset of migraines.

Symptoms
- Some children's eyes become sensitive; there may be pain behind the eyes, or they may experience an aura before the onset of their pain.
- The head pain can be an intense throbbing focused in one area or over one side of the head such that any movement of the head intensifies the discomfort.
- Often nausea and vomiting accompany migraine pain, so it is

important to take medication early, well before the nausea and
vomiting start.

- Some children experience rarer complicating symptoms, such as
numbness down one side of their body, as the head pain progresses.

Duration Migraine pain can last from minutes to hours and, in the extreme, for three to four days.

Triggers Some children have distinct food sensitivities—for example,
eating cheese or chocolate, or, for teens, drinking red wine may bring
on a migraine. Therefore, doing some detective work, such as keeping a
pain diary (see p. 86) to identify the triggers of each episode—and they
may include a number of factors, such as fatigue, diet, emotional distress, scholastic pressure, and peer stress—may lead to better headache
control.

Controlling the pain
- Learn what kind of stress triggers the migraine and how to minimize
or cope differently with this stress.
- Heeding and responding to early signs is a key step to gaining some
control of the pain.
- Learning not to fear the pain, responding promptly to the signals by
using relaxation and breathing techniques to reduce the pain and
tension, taking prescribed medication, and/or going to sleep in a
darkened room are some interventions that help.
- Sleep is often crucial to a full recovery from migraine pain.

For an excellent self-help program for headaches see "Help Yourself"
in the Recommended Resources.

Tension headaches These tend to be less dramatic than migraines, in that
there are no visual or body sensory disturbances, but they can be as bothersome and as distressing. Children often report that the pain feels like a
tight band around both sides of their head, lasting from part of an hour
to a few days. A seven-year-old girl explained: "When I get my headaches
my head feels hot and sore—it's like I'm wearing a pressure cap."

Possible causes
- Often the child's or teenager's neck muscles are tight and painful,
contributing to the build-up of pain and discomfort and perpetuating
the pain.
- The child's posture, or other sources of muscle strain, such as carrying

a heavy book bag or talking on the telephone by holding the phone with a raised shoulder, can contribute to the build-up of muscle tension that leads to a headache.

- Stress causes tension, which builds up to contribute to a tension headache. The stress can be physical, such as missing breakfast or exercising too much, or it can be emotional, such as feeling anxious before an exam or feeling the pressure of much to do within a short time.

Controlling the pain

- Using a pain diary (see p. 107A) to track when the headaches occur and what the child is doing before its onset can be very helpful in detecting which factors are stress triggers for the headaches. Once known, these triggers can be dealt with positively. Strategies for coping and changes in daily habits can help. These are detailed in the self-help program for headaches, *Help Yourself*, listed in Recommended Resources.
- Relaxation techniques are highly beneficial coping strategies in reducing and controlling tension headaches. Using breathing, relaxation, or imagery with relaxation and massage, the child or teen becomes aware of where in his forehead, scalp, neck and back there is tension and through these methods he can release the tension. As the tension is released, the pain diminishes.

Ten-year-old Matt, who regularly had tension headaches after school, used the imagery experience from his favorite vacation, snorkeling in Hawaii. Initially he needed 10 to 15 minutes to get his headache to diminish. After practicing his relaxation-imagery daily for ten days, he was able to ease the tension of school and release his headache from pain levels of 5 down to 0 within five minutes. He explained: "I'm so enjoying snorkeling again that my muscles relax and the pain just goes away!"

Since medications are not always effective for headaches, if children and their parents know about the flexibility and plasticity of pain systems, particularly in the quickly developing child, they may feel more confident turning to methods such as life-style changes, hypnosis, imagery, breathing, and relaxation. Even if there is a family history of headaches, these techniques can be very helpful in reducing the intensity, the duration, and even the frequency of the headaches. Appreciating more about how a pain signal becomes a pain experience opens up many more viable options for pain control and management.

Menstrual cramps (dysmenorrhea)

Symptoms Pain of menstruation is crampy or achy pain in the lower to mid-abdomen that can extend down the inner thighs and be experienced along with weakness, diarrhea, or nausea. During the first two years a girl's menstrual periods are usually not at all painful. Once ovulation begins, the levels of hormones increase in the bloodstream, leading to stronger contractions of the uterus and consequent discomfort and pain.

Incidence Menstrual cramping is experienced by about 40 to 60 percent of girls and women and is one of the leading causes of school absence for teenage high school girls.

Causes The pain and cramps, which usually occur on the first or second day of the girl's monthly menstruation, are caused when the muscles in the uterus (womb) contract and go into spasms, as the uterus works to expel the lining and blood that it has built up over the month. The uterine activity is mediated by a substance called prostaglandin; consequently, medication that inhibits prostaglandin activity, such as the NSAID (non-steroidal anti-inflammatory drug) group (see Chapter 7 for more information), is most effective for menstrual pain.

Coping with the pain How menstrual pain is interpreted and discussed with a teenage girl can often make the critical difference between whether she copes successfully with her pain or not. The key factor seems to be what the teenager has heard and learned from her mother. If she is told that her menstrual cramps are "the curse," she is likely to feel miserable, to feel that "girls have it rough," and to inhibit her activities. A teenage girl is more likely to cope well with the pain if she is told: "This pain is normal. It is a sign that your uterus is working properly, if a little too vigorously. It is a good sign that your uterus is strong and healthy, which is good to know if one day you want to be a mom."

Evidence suggests that cramps diminish after the first pregnancy and childbirth, owing to the stretching of the cervix. There is also some evidence that dysmenorrhea may decrease by the time women reach the age of 25. Both pieces of information may help your daughter move into a coping, rather than a victim, mode.

Controlling the pain Mild dysmenorrhea will often respond to a combination of rest and a hot water bottle or a hot bath. Stronger pain or cramps, however, require a visit to the physician and medication. Medication in the NSAID group, such as ibuprofen, decreases the pain as well as uterine contractions and is available over the counter in 200-mg tablets. Two tablets are usually recommended for the first dose. Again, the rule of thumb with pain is to take medication promptly at the first signs of pain. Use the recommended initial dose of medication to gain control of the pain; after the pain is well controlled, subsequent doses can be adjusted as needed.

Signs of unusual menstrual pain If your daughter appears very ill, has an unexplained fever, is unable to walk, or reports severe pain on one side of her lower abdomen, consult with your child's physician. Many girls do not volunteer to their doctor that they are having pain during menstruation. They may need some encouragement to help report this adequately so that they can cope better with this periodic discomfort.

Benign limb pain or "growing pains"

"Growing pains" is a term used to describe a child's brief and episodic limb pain that is not a symptom of an organic disorder and that occurs at night, often waking the child. In fact, the term "growing pains" is a misnomer, since the pain has nothing to do with growth. Rheumatologists believe that a better name for the condition is "benign limb pains of childhood." Despite the often frequent and severe nature of the pain, the children who experience this pain have no evidence of disease or dysfunction, nor do they develop any serious illness. A thorough medical examination should be performed to exclude such conditions as an unrecognized stress fracture, arthritis, cancer, or osteomyelitis.

Symptoms and causes Most often experienced by children aged four to nine, these pains are not yet well understood. The pain is usually a deep pain in the lower limbs. Whether the pain comes from muscle or bone (or both) is not clear. Usually the pain lasts a few minutes but is often so severe that the child is awakened from sleep and cries with the pain. The pain is almost always completely gone by next morning but may come back for several nights in a row. The pain can disappear for many weeks or months and then recur over the years, or never appear again. Many children with these intermittent leg pains are physically very active, and their pain may be the result of muscle tension caused by overexertion; when the muscles relax at night they can begin to hurt.

Controlling the pain

- Since the pain comes on quickly and can be scary, reassure your child by explaining that the muscles are aching from lots of activity.
- Invite your child to blow away the pain using regulated breathing, or with bubbles, as discussed previously.
- Discuss with your child which pain-relieving method—massage, medication, and/or heat—to use to help the pain go.
- Massage the limb gently and directly, easing, loosening, and warming the muscles. Massage for a minute or two is nearly always extremely helpful.
- If the pain is happening very frequently, a mild analgesic, such as acetaminophen, just before bedtime can help prevent the pain.
- Finally, heat in the form of a hot water bottle or a heating pad, or even just cuddling up in a sleeping bag, can keep the child's limbs warm enough to ensure a settled night. Avoid leaving a heating pad on a child's legs overnight.
- Consult with your child's physician if the limb pains are present in the morning or if your child has other symptoms, such as a fever, joint swelling, or difficulty in walking.

When the pain persists If the limb pains persist over time, as with the other recurring pain syndromes described above, it is important to address other factors, such as family distress, loss of or unhappiness with friends, or internal distress. Working with a mental health professional in tandem with the child's physician may be helpful. You should not fuss or overreact by, for example, taking the child into your bed at night. This can inadvertently lead to the persistence of the child's complaints of pain, as well as create discord between parents. When a distressed child is brought into the parent's bed at night, one parent tends to ends up sleeping in the spare bed, which can set up an unhealthy coping pattern for all involved.

MANAGING CHRONIC PAIN AT HOME

This topic deserves a book of its own; for further information, see Recommended Resources. This section focuses on strategies at home and at school to enable the child with chronic pain to re-engage in a normal life. A child's chronic pain can be deeply unsettling to the family and lead to frustration, fatigue, and continual readjustment for the child, brothers and sisters, and caregivers.

Strategies for dealing with pain

1. Establish a well-coordinated support system. Continually having to help a hurting child requires a great deal of reliable support for the adults and siblings in that child's life. Indeed, diseases such as cancer, AIDS, neuromuscular diseases, sickle cell disease, hemophilia, arthritis, and other persistent or progressive diseases are often managed in outpatient facilities of hospitals. The parents, however, especially the child's mother, are responsible for the primary and major care at home, providing the emotional and physical support, as well as dealing with the logistics of managing the home and frequent medical appointments. Therefore, the entire family, not just the child or teen who is living with the chronic pain condition or disease that causes pain, requires a well-coordinated support system composed of good home care support, such as a home care nurse, an excellent family physician or pediatrician, and a specialist, all of whom are available to be called. The support of specialized staff at a nearby hospital is also essential to keep your child as comfortable as possible at home and is best achieved by holding periodic team conferences with the hospital staff.

2. Allow other trusted people to take care of the child in pain at home. Bringing in another caregiver provides the child with someone different to relate to and gives parents a much needed change of scene. Whether this person is a babysitter, close family friend, relative, or respite nurse, you must take the time to review the key aspects of the child's care: what to do if the child's pain returns or worsens, where the important telephone numbers are, whom to call, where special medications are kept and how to administer them, how to talk to the child, and what pain-relieving method the child uses, such as TENS, an imagery tape, or a bag of frozen peas or heating pad. Chronic pain should not shut children off from relationships with friends and other key people, such as grandparents and close relatives.

3. Treat the pain promptly. As discussed in chapter 4, the nervous system itself changes, often becoming more sensitive and easily irritable as a result of the persisting pain signals. The pain can be as bad as the disease or trauma itself, although it is often not recognized as equally important in treatment. Jodi, a teenager in chronic pain, commented that in the provision of medical care, "First you should get the pain under control, then you treat the disease."

Sometimes, however, the treatment of pain goes hand in hand with that of disease. As is often true for arthritis or cancer pain, when the disease is promptly treated, the pain eases:

Tommy, a five-year-old, had been having leg pains for ten days and did not want to ride his bike or walk. Diagnosed with leukemia by his pediatrician, Tommy was treated as an outpatient in the oncology unit of the local children's hospital. He was started on chemotherapy as soon as the diagnosis was confirmed by the oncologist. Since the cause of his pain was a build-up of leukemia cells in the center of his bones, by treating the leukemia, the chemotherapy decreased the number of cells and his pain was relieved within 24 hours.

This rapid result does not occur with all conditions, however. Special attention and regular re-evaluation of the multi-method pain management program is frequently required.

4. *The child must become an authority on the pain in her body.* She must also be a key team member in the working alliance with the health professionals involved in her care.

- Time must be made to provide a full picture of why the child is experiencing pain, what the factors are that may modify the pain, and how the child can help to keep the pain manageable.
- Time must also be allowed for the child or teen to ask the many different questions that may arise as she lives with the pain. Understanding more about how pain works in the human body and in her body in particular can increase the child's control of situations that previously could have exacerbated the condition.
- More than in any other pain condition, the child in chronic pain must actively share authority with the health professionals in the regular care of her pain.

Helping Children with Chronic Pain Lead a Normal Life

Some children who are in chronic pain have a remarkable determination to re-engage in their normal activities. This determination can be a worry for parents: Should I let him go to school? Will this extra activity bring the pain back or intensify it? How will he manage if he gets worse? How can I enable him to lead as "normal" a life as possible with the condition he has? The rest of this chapter deals with these questions, drawing on research and our own experiences with families and in liaison with schools.

Parents who expect their child with a chronic illness to live as normally as possible may actually help their child experience less severe and disabling pain than those who do not set the same expectations for normality. Restricting a child's ability to play with friends, go to school, or continue with usual enjoyable childhood activities can feed into the child's feeling of not being well, or of being different and isolated, and can increase the child's pain. Creating a new definition of "normal" by maintaining what is possible and adapting activities and timetables helps the child with chronic pain to feel less "different" and to cope.

Counseling or joining a peer support group can help a child engage in normal life. Developing a buddy system with a neighborhood friend or with an older child who has a similar medical condition can also help. When the child is not experiencing pain, it is helpful to highlight what gives the child pleasure, fun, and a sense of achievement, rather than to dwell on how the pain eclipses her life. Being happier in other areas of her life will enable the child to cope, increasing self-esteem and reducing perceived pain.

HELPING THE FAMILY MANAGE WHEN A CHILD IS IN PAIN

The dynamics in the family change as the child's persistent or recurring pains keep him from school and normal play activities. His role in the household and with friends alters. He isn't able or willing to do many of the activities that he readily used to do. Family members have to adjust to these changes. Brothers and sisters can't play with him in the way they used to. He may require more rest and need the house to be quieter. Mealtimes may become more difficult as a result of having to prepare special foods for a picky eater or attempting to please everyone.

A major source of stress is that the extra attention that the child in pain receives often means less attention for other siblings in the family. Having a sick child at home affects every member of the family, even the dog, who may be disturbed by the strain or no longer get his walks. It often helps to talk about these adjustments in family meetings in which everyone, including the child in pain, has a say. Speaking without any interruption from others is a key rule to spell out in the beginning of the family talk; allow each member of the family to talk and be heard. Be sure to include yourself! Some questions parents might ask siblings of the sick child are:

- Since your brother or sister has been sick and in pain, a lot has changed at home—how do you feel about that?
- What do you miss most that we used to do in our family?

- What could Mom and Dad do that would make you feel happier, since it will be a while until he or she is well and pain-free again?
- What would you like to do with [the sibling in pain] even though he or she isn't yet his or her old self again?

Allow the conversation to roll from one sibling to another; ask the quieter ones if they agree or disagree with what is said. Decide what you as a family can do together or what each of you can do to bring the good feelings back into the family.

Returning your child to school

Some children say that the best part of being in sick or in pain is that they don't have to go to school. Be aware that long absences from school can be a factor in maintaining your child's pain. Your child may not want to give up the freedom of being at home and may fear returning to the classroom and all that work that has been missed. When the child's pain has begun to settle, use your judgment in encouraging him or her to attend school again.

School is a major focus of a child's social and academic activities. Children who cannot take part in school are being denied a major opportunity for age-appropriate social and work activities. Clinical experience and reports indicate that children experiencing pain who do not return to school early or as soon as they are able to find it increasingly difficult to reintegrate at a later time. So how do you go about enabling your recovering child to return to school?

A first move is to inform the school about what has happened to your child. Distribute some medical information to the teachers and school nurse and if there are many problems to address, such as the child's decreased energy and attention span or large amounts of missed work, organize a school-based team meeting, including the child. Taking these preliminary steps can be very helpful in setting up a suitable plan of action and gaining the cooperation of the entire team.

Work with the school to develop a plan for informing classmates why the child has been absent from school. Doing this early on, after the first absences, allows the classmates to keep the child in mind. Provide regular updates until the child is ready to return. At that time she may want to tell her story to the class and answer questions, or she may prefer to ignore her absence. These decisions about what, how much, and when to disclose her experiences must be left entirely up to her.

Some children like to be the center of attention. Other children or teens may prefer to have all the discussions and questions addressed before returning so that they can slip back into school without being made a "special case."

GUIDELINES TO EASE YOUR CHILD'S RE-ENTRY INTO SCHOOL

- Remind your child that he is the expert on his pain condition. As the expert, he can explain his pain to his friends so that they can gain a better understanding; sketches or diagrams can be very useful.
- Rehearse with your child what to say when asked, "Where have you been?" or "What happened to you?" Such preparation will help your child to gain some confidence in facing questions that may be embarrassing or to deal with any teasing.
- If you have access to school re-entry videotapes or materials made by the hospital, arrange to have these shown to the class before the child's return. With the aid of a therapist or nurse, the children can be encouraged to ask questions after the tape has been shown. The class may then be welcoming and considerate to the child on her return.
- Use a gradual re-entry approach to get your child back to school. For example your child can go for part of the day (the time of the day when the pain is least bothersome, such as the afternoon for a child with juvenile rheumatoid arthritis). Attending a few hours and gradually increasing school time eases school re-entry.
- Meet and discuss your game plan with the teacher so that there is support for your child's returning and remaining in class. Inform the teacher, the school nurse, and the class of the child's or teen's methods of coping with pain. You can also arrange with the teacher or school nurse to allow your child time to lie down if the pain recurs or to use helpful pain audio-tapes, medication, or walking to ease the pain.
- Keep the child's prescribed pain medication at the school so that it may be given at the required or needed times.
- Plan for predictable school problems, such as sports day or missed work, which may require extra-educational services.
- Track your child's daily school experiences. Social isolation is a miserable experience for any child, particularly a child in pain. Peer and social support for the child with recurring or chronic pain is central to the success of re-entry into school. Be proactive; discuss with your child his day-to-day experiences so that you are tracking his

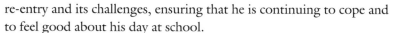

re-entry and its challenges, ensuring that he is continuing to cope and to feel good about his day at school.

- Confer with the school. Conferences with the teachers can be very helpful if there are problems that need ironing out. When the school staff members know your situation, they can be helpful allies in making your child's return to school as smooth as possible.
- Work with the school to maintain the child at school, even if attendance is irregular. The satisfaction of having a place to go, other than home and hospital, is very important for a child. It helps to develop social and work skills, nurtures self-esteem, and enables the child to feel like other children.

WHILE THE CHILD IS IN CLASS

Children with recurrent or chronic pain who want to remain at school learn to listen to their own bodies, to heed early warning signals that the pain is returning, and to take prompt action to prevent the pain from becoming worse. The three examples below show how children with different painful conditions heed their pain signals when they occur during class and take appropriate action to stay in school.

- A headache sufferer experiences an increase in neck muscle tension, and a throbbing in his temples begins. He does some neck rolls, and when the pain does not immediately ease, he excuses himself for a half hour to go lie down in the nurse's station and listen to a relaxation tape.
- A child with juvenile rheumatoid arthritis experiences mild achiness in her joints; she requests her medication from the teacher, stops walking around, and settles into a comfortable chair to rest and read a favorite book until the pain abates.
- A teenager with irritable bowel syndrome, loose stools, and lower abdominal cramps, excuses himself from the classroom, goes to the washroom to empty his bowels, then requests a hot water bottle from the first-aid teacher as he lies curled up on a bed visualizing his bowel easing, unwinding, and becoming smooth and relaxed. After 20 minutes he is able to return to the classroom.

Remind your child that she is the boss of her own body and that even if something dreadfully important is happening in class, it is more important that she help her pain to go away promptly. There is a place within the class for coping with pain, by breathing or relaxing. If moving eases the pain, your child should be able to leave the room and walk in the hall; if your child needs to lie down, it should be permissible to go to the nurse's station and lie down; if medication is needed, it must be promptly taken. If your child needs to call home, that too should be allowed. If the child's treatment options and plans for coping with her condition have been previously discussed, the teacher and the class will understand and support the needed steps.

Often children with persistent pain sleep poorly and consequently find it hard to sustain concentration in the classroom. This problem too should be shared with the teacher so that allowances can be made and alternatives provided. Our experience has been that when the child's medical condition is explained, the teacher has been exceptionally helpful in accommodating the child in pain. We have seen instances of great compassion: one grade four teacher brought in a special rocking chair from home so that her student with arthritis could rest and rock when her joints began aching. At the same time she could continue to hear what was going on in the classroom without feeling isolated in the sick room.

Conclusion

Children in acute pain, recurring pain, or persistent chronic pain can be treated and managed at home by parents, caregivers, and in some cases, themselves. Children who experience recurring pain need to become an active part of their treatment plan. These children or teens need support to reconnect and re-engage in their social and school life, since outside involvement with friends, activities, and learning plays a crucial role in promoting recovery and well-being.

CHAPTER 9

Visiting the Doctor

THIS SIX-YEAR-OLD BOY'S first response to visiting his doctor contains everything that parents want to avoid: "I heard my mom say we soon had to go to the doctor and I'd heard a lot of bad things about the doctor so I hid in my cupboard, but she started yelling and getting real mad so I came out" (Ross and Ross).

What an unfortunate experience for both child and parent! It would have been better if the child had been able to:

- Know his doctor and to have had good experiences with him or her well before the age of six;
- Understand why he was going and what would happen in the doctor's office; and
- Discuss his concerns or fears with his mom or the doctor.

It would also have been better if the child's mother had not lost her temper and had to coerce her child to go to the doctor.

Why Children Fear Going to the Doctor

Why are some children reluctant to visit their physician? The majority of these children say they fear experiencing pain or having a needle. Generally, physicians don't want children to experience pain in their consulting rooms. They would like children to feel comfortable and relaxed. This can be achieved even when pain brings the child in to see the doctor, and parents can play a pivotal role by preparing and coaching their children to handle pain. If an office's schedule overrides a child's need for more preparation or explanation, the parent must act as advocate for the child, voicing on behalf of the child what needs must be met or what fears need to be addressed.

Many family doctors and pediatricians do their best to make their offices a pain-free zone. Minor surgeries may be done in the hospital, or laboratory technicians may collect a child's blood in an outside laboratory. Some doctors rely on public health nurses or their own nurse to give immunizations in a designated treatment area. Many physicians, especially in small communities, must stitch lacerations, treat fractures and other injuries, or give inoculations in the surgery room attached to their consulting room. Parents can do a great deal to ease their children's anxieties in all these situations. If their concerns, pain, and distress are not sensitively handled, the doctor's office can become a place where children learn fear and mistrust.

Doctor As Teacher

Did you know that the term "doctor" comes from the Latin *docere*, and means "teacher"? A visit to the doctor demonstrates that we can look at, listen to, understand, and manage our bodies' symptoms and pains. The doctor's office provides a learning opportunity; it is a place to bring concerns and explore ways of maintaining one's well-being and good health.

The learning starts early. From birth most babies have been "checked over." They have had their hearts listened to, their ears looked at, and their eyes examined, and later, they have been asked to do the famous "Aaah" for a throat examination. A baby does not "remember" these very early experiences in the strict sense of being able to recall them. Research suggests, however, that from six months onwards a child may "record" the experience of going to the doctor, and so the doctor's office becomes a familiar environment.

As children get older, their visits to the doctor become a forum for receiving information about their bodies and how they will grow. Children learn over successive visits not only that their bodies show signs when something isn't well but that there is someone apart from their parents who can look at these signs, diagnose what they mean, and tell them what to do to get well again. The best arrangement is for the same person to see your child each visit—a family doctor, nurse practitioner, or pediatrician—so that your child develops some degree of comfort and trust.

Start with well-baby visits to maintain your baby's good health and determine feeding, sleeping, and growth patterns. These visits can also provide an excellent way for all of you—parents and child—to become comfortable with your family doctor. It is best to find a doctor with whom you can develop a trusting relationship. In times of illness and stress, one of the first people to whom you will turn for help is your family doctor. If you trust him or her without hesitation, you will transfer this trust to your children.

Some Guidelines for Selecting a Doctor for Your Family

The relationship comes first and foremost. Trust your instincts. Ask yourself these questions:

- Do I like and feel comfortable with this person?
- Can I talk to this person?
- Does this person listen closely to what I say?
- Does this person take prompt and responsive action?
- Does this person seem thorough?
- Do I sense a growing trust with this person?
- How does this person handle my child or baby?
- How does my child respond to this person?
- Is this person respectful of my child?
- Does this person talk directly, explain procedures, and listen to my child's responses?

The overriding principle behind the above guidelines is that a truly cooperative partnership should be established between an informing physician and an aware parent and child. Your doctor is there to assist you, teach you, guide you, and inform you. You and your child have many rights. These include the right to ask questions, to check procedures, to request more information, to voice your concerns, and to know that these will be heard and respected. If you do not feel right about your physician, do not feel you have to stay loyal simply because you have known him or her for a long time. Even a doctor with the best reputation may not be the best one for you and your child.

After you have found a doctor with whom you feel good, stay with this person. Do not doctor-shop. It is much better for both your family and the doctor to have this relationship develop over time. Your doctor will learn to appreciate you, will come to know your family and circumstances, and will be better able to make recommendations based on that knowledge. It is also helpful for you to know your doctor's office practices, including arrangements for evening, weekend, and holiday coverage and emergencies. You will then know what to do if your child becomes ill or is in pain during the night—when it is difficult to think clearly.

Preparation for Visiting the Doctor

If your child is ill or in pain, you may take her in for an unscheduled visit. Always tell your child before you set out where the two of you are going. Don't spring the news en route—"Oh, by the way, before we go to McDonald's, we'll just stop by to see the doctor." If your child has apprehensions about going to the doctor, tricking her into a visit will not allay those fears; it will probably increase them and cause your child to distrust your intentions.

No matter how anxious you are, always prepare your child, whatever his age. Discuss the purpose of the visit on the day you intend to go or, if your child is older, a day or two before. You know what will work best for your child and what time frame and information will not arouse anxiety. Take the time to answer any questions your child might have and discuss what could make this visit go well. This team work will give your child the chance to become mentally, emotionally, and physically prepared for the visit.

The visit does not need to be "worked to death," however. With an 18-month-old toddler, the conversation could go like this:

Parent: Poor baby, your nose is running. You're not feeling well, are you? You're pulling on your ear. Is your ear hurting? Is it sore?

Toddler: (whimpering and distressed)

Parent: We're going to visit Dr. Rogers to see what's happening in your ears, because they're bothering you. Dr. Rogers will take a peek into your ears with a little light and see what is going on inside. She'll also ask you to open your mouth like this (opens mouth) to see if your throat is sore too. Is your throat sore? What toy and books shall we take with us for our visit? Let's be sure to take your bottle and your blankey and some bubbles.

Don't tell your child that "the doctor is not going to hurt you." First, it introduces the idea of hurt, and your child may not have even given it a thought. Once hurt is mentioned, the notion is planted. Your child will associate your doctor with hurt, which may make your child fearful. Second, you don't know what the doctor is going to do; therefore, if pain is not an issue, it is best not to bring it up.

If pain will occur as part of the visit, it is important not to lie to your child. This is a sticky situation; the question about how to prepare a child for a painful procedure can be as tough on health care professionals as it is on parents. We don't want to hurt our children, and conveying that something will cause them pain makes us uncomfortable. Often, however, we cause more pain and anxiety when we try to spare those fears. By avoiding the truth, we also avoid the opportunity for the child to be prepared and feel supported.

If you don't know whether it is going to hurt or not, be candid and say, "I don't know, but we'll find out." If you know it is going to hurt, here are some things you can do and say:

- Tell the truth with compassion: "It may hurt."
- In the same breath, convey your belief that your child can deal with the pain—that the pain is not bigger than she is.
- Then mobilize your child's courage and ability to cope: "You may be surprised how little it does bother you, like the time that . . ." (Draw on an earlier example of when he coped better than he expected to.)
- Don't get caught up in discussing the small size of the needle, or how few vials of blood will be drawn, since these are details you have no control over.
- Be calm; provide reassurance and helpful, practical suggestions. Emphasize that the two of you will work as a team to do the things that will make the experience go smoothly.

If you do these things, your child will be better able to take in the tough news, will trust you, and will not feel immobilized by anxiety.

Here is an example of how a pre-teen or teenager's question "Do you think it will hurt?" could be dealt with:

Parent: Having an injection may cause some discomfort—that's why it's important to use a coping technique to make it easier. What would you like to do to help yourself? Do you want to squeeze my hand, count to ten, or do some deep relaxing breathing?

Teen: I guess . . . breathing.

Parent: That's what we used when you were born. Breathing helped me a great deal. Your needle won't seem to take nearly as long! Remember, your breathing will blow the pain and tension out. When you deliberately relax like that you'll not feel the pain as much. It works—I know from my own experience.

Alex, a physically active six-year-old, fell off a climbing structure into the gravel below, gashing both his chin and his forehead. This is how Darby, a mother of three, prepared her child for the unexpected visit to their doctor's surgery. Suppressing her own distress and shock at the gravel lodged in the open bloody wounds on her child's face, she held an ice pack on both forehead and chin until a neighbor brought her car around. Then the following exchange took place:

Darby: It's really good that we're off to see Dr. Baldwin because he'll put some freezing medicine in so that we can clean this stuff out.

Alex: Will it hurt, Mom?

Darby: Well, it may, but probably no more than it's hurting now. And you're doing well right now. We'll do our best to make you comfortable. Let's take Teddy; he always helps. Dr. Baldwin may give you some pain medicine because you may have to have some stitches. I'll be with you all the time. It'll be okay. Your body knows how to heal.

WHAT TO TAKE ALONG

Even though you may have a scheduled appointment, waiting longer than you expected is all too common in a doctor's waiting room. Take along some of your child's favorite toys and books. If your child is in pain or discomfort, take along one of the therapeutic aids listed in chapter 6, such as ice, a favorite storybook, a warm bottle, or bubbles, and if you are able, include a treat as a surprise distraction.

Older children are particularly neglected in this way. Parents often say "She's eleven now; she won't need anything." Remember, even a confident eleven-year-old can behave like a clinging six-year-old if she is fearful or in pain. Throwing a few familiar items together, such as the comics, your child's current novel, Lego, or a Transformer before you fly out the door is well worth the extra minute it takes. You'll be able to hold your child's attention, keep your child calm and focused, and make the visit to the doctor less stressful.

When Old Fears Are Revived

For children with persistent medical problems, visiting the doctor conjures up memories of previous hospitalizations and painful treatments. These children are not novices. The doctor's visit was often the prelude to these intensive treatments, and therefore visiting the doctor may carry another layer of fear. Nine-year-old Josh, who has a history of unusual cardiac problems, always rigorously grills his mother when she informs him that they have to go visit their doctor. You'll notice Josh's controlled but evident anxiety in their recorded conversation, while his mom attempts to ally his fears.

Josh: Why do I have to see him?

Mom: It's just a routine check, Josh. Nothing to worry about.

Josh: But what is he going to do? I hate going!

Mom: It's the usual, Josh. You remember — blood pressure, pulse, listening to your heart and lungs. You do fine with it every time. You know what to expect.

Josh: But why now?

Mom: It's June. We go every two months. The last visit was April. Josh, what are you worried about now?

Josh: Last time I ended up in hospital, remember? I had blood work and that awful catheterization.

Mom: I don't think that will happen this time. But I do know it was pretty hard on you last time. You're worried about going through that again. Remember that the results were good from that last session. This is just our ordinary routine check.

In this situation, it is important not to belittle or play down your child's fears. For example, a common but counterproductive response might be: "Don't be silly, there's nothing to be afraid of!" ["You wanna bet!" thinks the child. "You don't have to go through it—I do!"] Another common unhelpful response is: "Be a big boy and make your mother proud!"

While being sympathetic, guard against feeding your child's fears (as occurred with with Hailey on p. 67). This can be achieved by:

- Understanding the nature of your child's particular fears reminding your child of what routinely occurs;
- Recalling how she usually copes; and
- Deciding what you can do to help.

The Doctor's Examination

The physical examination is in the doctor's hands. It is largely up to your doctor to be inventive and playful and make the examination as smooth as possible. Many are very kind and gentle and, where possible, give the child choices and control. Experienced doctors work quickly and deftly, knowing that time is short with wriggly, restless children. You can support this process.

Your doctor may choose to examine your toddler or preschooler on your lap. This is preferable for many children. It maintains a warm sense of security and allows you to comfort and coach your child. This is also a good way to begin an examination until the child is able to sit unaided on the examining table. This may occur at any age but most commonly occurs about three or four years of age, depending on your child's level of independence and confidence, as well as what needs to be examined.

BUNNIES IN THE EAR

Certain parts of the examination can be frightening to a child. For example, it is often very upsetting for toddlers to have their ears or other orifices poked and prodded. Holding still is also very difficult to do. Imagination and a sense of play help in these situations. On one occasion, a seasoned and playful pediatrician told a squirming 2 1/2-year-old with a possible middle ear infection: "Hold very very still so that I can take a close look and find the bunny rabbit that jumped into your ear. That's great! Oh! I can see him; he's jumping over the fence. Hold still! Oh! He's gone across to the other ear. Quickly, let me look in the other ear. That's it! Ah, I've found him, do you know what he's doing? He's wiggling his nose at me!"

The pediatrician rattled this off as he deftly completed his examination. The child sat wide-eyed and remarkably still for the minute that was needed.

Doctors have remarked that having something fun to do with the child often takes the monotony out of these routine procedures. Like children, adults too are capable of doing more than one thing at a time. If you know your young child's current favorite animal or current interest, mention this to your doctor. You could also prompt your child to tell the doctor about the book she is reading, or the school trip she went on. This can make the examination more personal and interesting.

Older children in pain may also like some contact from a parent during their physical examination, such as holding their hand, stroking their forehead, or even making direct eye contact across the room. Some children feel quite vulnerable during a physical examination. Your presence may make it easier. If an older child prefers to see the doctor on his own, or to be examined without you there, however, respect his wishes.

If present, parents can be invaluable allies for the doctor. You can, for example:

- Interpret what the doctor is saying or doing so that your child understands.
- Encourage your child to cooperate.
- Distract your child's attention when she becomes bored or restless. A mobile, mirror, picture in the room, or stories from memory can all be used.
- Prompt your child to speak up for herself.

RESTRAINING: THE PROS AND CONS

Generally, it is preferable that your child not be restrained for a physical examination. Cooperation and learning how to manage during a medical examination are always better. If restrained, children remember and tend to become fearful and panicky about future examinations, and it is more difficult to re-establish trust. If your child is not cooperative, it is crucial that you not resort to threats. The worst threat that we have heard is: "If you don't sit still, the doctor will give you a shot!" Doctors and nurses cringe when they hear this. Most will promptly deny it and say something comforting to the child. Instead of using the threat of pain as coercion, use humor and, if you are desperate, bribe with a treat. All of these methods are acceptable to gain your child's cooperation.

There are times when explanations, coaching, or bribery are counterproductive. Infants or toddlers, particularly if they are ill, have a difficult time settling, even on a parent's lap. A parent shouldn't be reluctant to firmly and calmly steady a child's hand or support a wiggling head to assist a safe and thorough exam, especially of the ears and throat. In these brief situations explanation and reassurance are of no benefit. They may even feed the child's fear and resistance, and increase everyone's anxiety. When a child has "lost it," it is hard to regain cooperation. Intervening before that time is essential.

A restraining hug for 15 seconds will not be traumatic for a young child. In these short examinations, many family physicians prefer the child to be held by a parent. During an arm or leg injection, hugging containment takes this form: the child sits on the parent's lap facing the parent, with the parent's arms around the child, keeping one of the child's arms free for the injection. For a leg injection, the child sits on the parent's lap with her back against the parent's chest. One leg, tucked in between the parent's knees, is held for the immunization; the other leg is free. This type of brief restraint is also useful for an ear examination, since the parent can subdue the child's flailing arms and stabilize the child's head. A parent's hugging containment is a brief restraint and prevents further escalation of distress. It should not be used for longer procedures, since it is hard to maintain the compassionate interaction inherent in the hug. If held longer, it may no longer be experienced by the child as loving but as coercive.

With older children and teenagers, restraint is only an option in life-threatening and emergency situations. The key to achieving cooperation is to respect the teen and provide whatever choices are possible, such as setting a time: "When do you feel better about going, this morning or in the afternoon? I'll see what is available."

THE CHILD AS SPOKESPERSON FOR THE PAIN

Children need to be encouraged to speak for themselves, relating how their bodies feel, where they hurt, and how much they hurt. You might use one of the scales in chapter 5 with your child to measure the different degrees of pain. Children can be encouraged to tell

- When the pain started
- What makes it worse
- What makes it feel better
- What makes the pain stop entirely.

Most doctors will address your child directly. If the questions are directed to you, and you know your child is capable of answering them, simply defer to your child, encouraging him to answer. This sends an important message and establishes that you know your child is capable of being the authority of her body. The earlier this process is established, the better it is for your child's developing sense of self.

THE PARENT AS INTERPRETER AND FACILITATOR

As a parent, you are often attuned to the subtleties of your child's behavior. You know how to read your child's signals, interpret your child's unspoken reactions, and clarify what your child is attempting to convey. As interpreter, you can reword what the doctor is saying when it is clear to you that your child doesn't fully understand the doctor's words. For example, a seven-year-old became visibly distressed when her doctor said that she was going to take her blood pressure. Knowing her daughter's fear of needles, her mother immediately added, "Dr. Sandy is just measuring the pressure around your arm, Jenny. That tells your blood's pressure. It doesn't hurt. She's not going to take out any blood!"

Medical jargon can lead to misunderstandings. It is always preferable to use words for bodily functions that children know, rather than polysyllabic or medical words. Many families don't use complex words like "diarrhea" or "constipation" with their children. A doctor may ask if a child is constipated, and wanting to be pleasing and cooperative, the child may say yes without understanding what being constipated means. More and more families and doctors realize that simple words like "pooing" and "peeing" are easier for children to understand. "Genitals" is another common term that is not known by younger children. Tell your doctor what the family's words are for defecation, urination, anus, vulva, and penis so that the doctor and your child can talk the same language.

COMMON PROCEDURES AT THE DOCTOR'S

Immunizations, lacerations, and infections of the throat, ears, chest, and gastrointestinal and urinary tracts are common reasons for visiting a family doctor. All of these conditions can be painful.

Immunization

Immunizations are the most effective way of preventing common childhood infections such as diphtheria, whooping cough, tetanus, polio, meningitis, measles, mumps, and rubella. For a healthy baby, it is also the first experience of the pain of an injection. Immunizations are given in the thigh muscle in babies and toddlers and in the arm in older children. These injections are given at 2 months, 4 months, 6 months, 12 months, 18 months, and 5 years of age, often just before the child starts kindergarten. They are painful and unpleasant, and they may leave local irritation or swelling that may feel tender and sore for a few days.

How parents can help
- Use EMLA®, the cream local anesthetic, described on p. 178 on the leg or arm site 60 to 90 minutes before the immunization. The medication creates a numb area where the cream has been placed and the child will not feel pain when the skin is punctured.
- Give your child the recommended dose of acetaminophen half an hour *before* the pain occurs. This allows time for the medication to be absorbed into the system and to become active, minimizing the pain and discomfort during and after the injection. Pediatricians recommend two subsequent follow-up doses, at four and eight hours, and if needed every four hours up to 24 hours after the injection. Pain medication given around the clock will prevent the pain from recurring if the injection site is still red or painful a day or two following immunization.
- Use one of your cool aids (see p. 126), such as an Ouch Mouse, a cool cloth, or a frozen sponge, to reduce the inflammation.
- Ensure that your child gets extra sleep.

Immunizations do sting sharply. Even with EMLA®, there may be some stinging. Be prepared, therefore, to provide immediate comfort and soothe your infant or child during and after the procedure.

Soothing your baby
- Hold your baby yourself during the injection. The experience of the needle is shock enough; your baby doesn't need to be in a stranger's arms as well.
- Use breast or bottle feeding. If your baby will accept the nipple, it is a speedy way of allowing your baby to rapidly regain familiar security.
- Rapid moving and rocking can also be an effective soother, at 50 to 60 beats a minute (see p. 135). This strong rhythmic rocking, also provided by women who carry their babies on their backs while working, regulates the child's crying and breathing patterns. The baby can then be given the breast or bottle and further soothed.

For your preschooler For preschoolers, preparing your child the day before or the day of the immunization is enough. For an explanation of immunization, you could say something along these lines or select parts of the section below:

Before you can go to school, we have to make sure your body is protected against diseases like polio and whooping cough. The best protection is to help your body make special police officers, called "antibodies," against these diseases. Your body can do this when you are given an immunization, because it gets your body's protection system (the immune system) to make special police officers inside your body to protect you.

You had five immunization injections when you were a baby, and this is the last for many years. So what do you think will help you handle it without being too bothered? We could do some blowing to make sure the hurt doesn't hang in longer than it should. Let's practice some bubble blowing; that always helps.

The use of EMLA® as part of the preparation for the five-year-old's immunization is highly recommended, particularly for children who are needle phobic. This topical anesthetic will, however, take the deep muscle pain away, and children may still require acetaminophen for any persistent pain and limb tenderness.

Ear infection

Otitis media, infection of the middle ear, is one of the more common painful infections of early childhood. Babies may, but do not always, "tell" you, by tugging an ear lobe or crying more than usual, that they have an ear infection. Pain is a direct result of the infection, so the best treatment is to seek medical attention. The pain can be treated with an age-appropriate dose of acetaminophen (see Table 8.1 on p. 180) until your child's ear is examined and decisions about treatment are made; antibiotics have been the treatment of choice for ear infections. When the infection is under control, the pain should rapidly recede. Until then, the pain can be controlled and relieved with around-the-clock four-hour doses of acetaminophen.

Cuts

The pain with a cut or laceration is greatest at the time when the injury occurs. Thereafter, the site will be very tender, throbbing, and sensitive. Seeing an open wound with flowing blood is traumatic, but this trauma should not be magnified by a parent's anxiety. Reactions such as "Oh my! Doctor, what are we going to do? This is terrible!" make the situation far worse. We know that the parent's attitude is pivotal in how the child responds to this injury. Physicians have remarked that parents who calmly ask: "Do we need any stitches, or will a Band-aid do?" generally have children who are equally calm.

Once anxiety takes over, it is very difficult to rescue the situation. When overwhelmed by fears, a child finds it hard to listen to the doctor, take in new information, or hold still for stitching. A very anxious child can benefit from calm talking, soothing touch, and, if needed, anxiety medication. Physicians commonly use a swab soaked with a topical spray called TAC (tetracaine, adrenaline, and cocaine), or an injectable local anesthetic called lidocaine or xylocaine, which, if in a buffered form, diminishes the sting as it is infused into the wound. Within two to five minutes the local anesthetic will numb the area and provide adequate pain relief for suturing lacerations.

Abdominal pain

Abdominal pain is extremely common in childhood. The pain may be acute (with sudden onset), or it may be a persistent, grumbling type of pain. The causes for both acute and chronic abdominal pain include indigestion, constipation, appendicitis, and gastrointestinal infections and diseases, as well as worry, conflict at home, or stress at school. In the latter situations, children's abdominal pains are analogous to adult's headaches: the pain is real, but there is no disease or infection.

Rather, the head or the abdomen is sensitive and responds to distress and internal pressure.

If your child complains of abdominal pains, she should be thoroughly assessed and given a physical exam by a physician. After serious medical concerns have been ruled out, the history of the child's pain, which the physician will elicit by questioning you and your child, often becomes more important than the physical examination. Remember, your child can experience genuine, persistent abdominal pain even though your physician may not reach a clear diagnosis. Other factors, such as fears and seemingly irresolvable worries (the brain's contribution), can maintain pain in a sensitive organ like the stomach. The child's or teen's abdominal pain is real and deserves thoughtful and thorough attention and treatment.

If the abdominal pains persist and disrupt your child's life, your physician is likely to track the pain over successive appointments, questioning your child and listening carefully to his or her concerns to determine which triggers are causing the pain. Your leads and support for this exploratory process can help the physician make a clearer assessment and treatment decision. Sometimes you may be referred to a gastrointestinal specialist for further medical investigations. Often the continuation of abdominal pains indicates that a broader-based pain management therapy is needed and that pain medication by itself may not be helpful. Your physician may refer your child for psychotherapy, nutritional evaluation and dietary changes, educational assessments (if there are school concerns), or family therapy. All these interventions help reduce the pain and internalized pressure that the child may be feeling.

Abdominal pain can require an examination of the genitalia, as well as a rectal exam, to exclude hernias, for example, or testicular problems. Children naturally feel shy, and many have been schooled about sexual abuse and so are particularly sensitive to having their panties down or their penis examined. In the case below, the doctor eases this nine-year-old boy's fears by addressing both him and his parent together. The parent helps the child feel safer by adding his consent:

Dr. Charles (to the child, while looking occasionally at the parent): So that we can figure out what will help you with this pain, I'll have to carefully check your whole tummy as well as your bottom. First I'm going to check your whole tummy, then I'll check your penis, because sometimes it can cause tummy pains, and then I'll do a rectal exam, which means I'll put a little vaseline on my glove and check with my finger right inside your bottom. This may feel a little weird, but it doesn't usually hurt. I'll begin at your tummy and go all the way down. Okay?

Parent: It's okay, Jay, Dr. Charles is just feeling different parts of your body. He is allowed to do that because he's figuring out what we should do about your pain. I'm here with you. It'll be okay.

The parent's reassurance and support can make this delicate examination easier.

Headaches

Tension headaches and migraines are more common in children and teenagers than is often recognized, and they are frequently caused by fatigue and stress. (See p. 198 for a discussion of children's headaches and how best to assess and manage them at home.) Most headaches are benign, but your child's physician will examine the child neurologically and ascertain the history of the pain to exclude the possibility of a brain tumor.

Physicians often encourage parents and the child to consider what factors in the child's life may trigger the child's pain. For example, children with a demanding schedule of extracurricular activities after a busy school day and homework are commonly prone to headaches. Teens who don't eat regularly or whose sleep schedule is irregular can experience headaches related to hypoglycemia and fatigue, respectively. Children with chronically blocked sinuses can experience sinus headaches, which throb and may feel like tension headaches. Draw your physician's attention to any patterns you have observed, such as the days, or time of day, that your child's headaches tend to occur, and the circumstances under which they occur, and what you suspect the triggers are for these headaches. A pain diary (see p. 107A) can be helpful in doing this detective work.

Analgesics are not a satisfactory long-term solution if the headaches occur daily or are triggered by regular conflict in the home, among friends, or at school. Often your physician will ask the child a range of questions to encourage her to reflect on whether these aspects of her life may be contributing to her headaches and how better to deal with these problems. A pain management program may be recommended (for details of an excellent program called *Help Yourself*, see Recommended Resources) and the physician may refer you and your child for psychotherapy and training in pain management.

Taking a throat swab from a child's sore throat

It is usually hard for children to open their mouths wide enough for a swab culture to be taken from the throat. This is particularly true if your child has experienced this procedure before and resists. You can reassure the child that the procedure won't hurt, that it might feel a little strange, but that it will not be painful. Here is a useful technique for preparing your child for this procedure: Ask your child to cup his hand; then spread his fingers open. Using the thumb as the lower jaw and the fingers as the upper jaw, show how wide the child's jaw needs to open. Stroke the palm in a manner similar to taking a swab. Separate the thumb from the fingers to wide open, showing the child how smoothly and gently he can open the mouth. Have the child do this. Show how the swab goes in and then explain that the swab will show the doctor which germs are making the child's throat hurt.

Because they fear the worst, some children will scream no matter what you do; others will stall, argue, or try to give reasons why they can't open their mouths wider. Some children may have had traumatic experiences before. Tell the child that "we will help you do this." Bargaining and bribery are acceptable in these situations—suggesting a treat at McDonald's, for example. Threats are never helpful; they increase the child's fears, worsen the situation, and make the next throat swab even more traumatic.

Urinalysis

A urine analysis is often required if a child experiences pain on urinating or a kidney or bladder infection is suspected. To urinate on demand is difficult even for adults. If a urine sample is needed, collect the specimen at home in a sterile jar supplied by the lab. It is difficult for children to urinate in an unfamiliar setting under stressful circumstances, particularly if urinating is painful. Home is more comfortable and private. Finding it difficult to produce on demand, some children have come up with ingenious solutions in laboratory washrooms: running tap water into the urine cup or scooping water from the toilet bowl after urinating into it! The same principles apply to collecting stool specimens—there is no place like home.

Pelvic exams for girls

Pelvic examinations are not done on girls who are not sexually active unless there are strong indications, such as persistent lower abdominal or pelvic pain, of sexual abuse or rape. A rectal exam may be done instead of a vaginal exam, or an exam may be done under general anesthetic, if appropriate. Most physicians do not even do a pelvic exam when giving birth control pills to a teen who is not yet sexually active.

When a pelvic exam is medically indicated in a sexually active teen, a complete explanation before the examination is helpful and needed. Some physicians will explain what they are doing as they do the exam. This can be very reassuring. If carefully done, this examination may feel strange and uncomfortable, but generally it is not painful as long as there isn't any pelvic trauma.

Teens who are sexually active sometimes prefer having a girlfriend accompany them for a gynecological check-up. If an older child or teenager comes in with a parent, she should be asked alone whether or not she wants her mother present during the exam. Some girls like their mothers to be present during their first pelvic exam. Others feel more comfortable if their mother isn't present but may feel guilty voicing this preference. Mothers should allow their daughters to freely choose. A pelvic exam should never under any circumstances be coerced or forced. A parent can act as an advocate in these circumstances.

Even though the doctor's office may be associated with pain, the majority of children are able to see this experience in a positive light. When the parent acts as interpreter, facilitator, and advocate for the child in the early years, the child learns over time how to speak up about any health concerns and develops a comfortable relationship with and trust of the physician.

CHAPTER 10

Visiting the Dentist

The dentist. I guess you could say that all children have a fear of them at one time or another. Who wouldn't? You're sitting in a chair, mouth wide open, and a person is sticking a drill in your mouth.

— JEREMY, AGE 14

FEAR OF PAIN AT THE DENTIST'S office is more of a problem than pain itself. But anxiety increases pain, and if children's fears are neglected or dismissed, they can magnify any discomfort and make good pain management difficult to achieve. Unlike hospitals, however, today's dental offices routinely address fears and general anxieties as thoroughly as they manage pain. Pain prevention and control is a priority in dental procedures and dentists tend to be well trained in pain management. They are taught to take active steps to prevent pain, rather than treating it after it arises and has begun to unnerve the child.

Over the last two decades the training of dentists, and consequently the practice of dentistry in North America, has changed dramatically. Dental schools have included the management of pain and anxiety as an essential part of their training curriculum, years ahead of either nursing schools or medical schools.

Whereas many adults have unpleasant memories of going to the dentist as a child, most children today are quite blasé about going for their routine dental visits. A child needs only one negative experience such as beginning to gag and the dentist becoming impatient, for the child to develop fears of further pain and a strong desire to avoid any more dental work.

This chapter examines how to choose a suitable dentist for your child, how to prepare your child for a visit to the dentist, and how to cope with a visit (whether or not pain is a part of the dental visit). It covers how dentists deal successfully with pain, describes the current position on practices such as general anesthesia and sedation, and explains how to handle painful and traumatic dental emergencies.

Before the Visit

Today the focus in dentistry is on preventing dental problems. Many dentists like to see a child by the age of one year, or shortly after the child's first teeth appear, followed by regular six-month visits to monitor the eruption of the child's teeth and to identify cavities in their early stages. These visits also provide regular and pain-free opportunities for the child to become familiar with the dentist, the dental staff, and the environment of the office.

CHOOSING THE RIGHT DENTIST

Not all dentists enjoy working with children. Some dentists become exasperated when children are fearful and uncooperative. Others may feel guilty or unsure about how to relate to anxious children. Some dentists feel uncomfortable having parents in the office with the child. Since it is desirable that this relationship, like your relationship with your family physician, be a long-term one, it is worth taking the time to find a dentist with whom you feel comfortable, who is known to be competent, and above all, who works well with children.

GUIDELINES FOR CHOOSING A DENTIST

- Do the dental office and dentist have policies and an atmosphere that suit your own philosophy? For example, are parents allowed in the office during their child's dental work? Some offices discourage this practice. It is worth discussing.
- Do the dentist and dental staff listen closely to what you say about your child?
- Do they take prompt, responsive, and thorough action?
- Do they talk directly to your child?
- How does your child respond to them?
- Do they explain the procedures ahead of time, involve your child in a practical way, and allow for questions?
- Do they encourage your child to take care of his teeth?
- Do they give the child the invitation to show "stop" with a hand so that the child has partial control and feels more comfortable?

PREPARING FOR THE DENTAL VISIT

After you have selected a good dentist for your child, not much preparation is required for a visit. Telling your toddler or preschool child the day of the visit, or your school-aged child a day or two beforehand, that you are going to the dentist may be enough, depending on the child's individual needs. Preparing your preschooler or school-aged child can be done in a matter-of-fact way: "We're going to see your new dentist. I've chosen this person because your cousin goes there and likes her. We need to make sure that your teeth are growing well and are healthy, and that you are brushing and flossing correctly. Your new dentist will be able to tell and will help you learn if you're not doing it quite right."

Some parents may be anxious about the procedures that need to be done to their child and about how the child will respond. These anxieties affect how the child anticipates the dental experience. If you feel negative about dental visits or have had negative experiences yourself in the dental chair, be aware of how you talk about the dentist. Children are very sensitive to the emotional tone of what parents say. If your dread or distrust shows even subtly, this may influence your child. One way of dealing with this predicament with a child five years or older is to be candid with the child. You could, for example, say something along these lines: "When I was a child, some dentists didn't know about how to handle children as well as they do today. My dentist certainly didn't have good ways to make me feel comfortable. So I had bad experiences then, and I have some left-over bad feelings about those times. But now with Dr. Goodheart, I don't have bad experiences anymore. She's kind and makes everything go pretty easily. So I'm pleased that you are going to see her. You'll find it new and interesting, and it'll be very different for you than it was when I was a child."

If your anxieties about dental work persist, speak to your dentist, *out of your child's hearing*. Explain that you had negative dental experiences and that you don't want this to happen to your child. Ask for guidance about what needs to be conveyed to your child and what words you can use to help build your child's confidence. These actions will go a long way towards building a bond between you and the dentist and will also help your child.

The Dental Examination

At the dentist's office you can help make the visit successful by being calm and supportive, both of your child and of the dental team as they proceed. A parent who gives instructions during the examination that conflict with those given by the dental staff can confuse the child and irritate the staff. If the team does not understand or handle your child well, however, you need to speak on behalf of your child. Conversely, if all is going well, it is best to take a back seat. The dental team tends to have a finely tuned, fairly rapid routine, which includes their own child-oriented language for the dental equipment and procedures.

DENTAL TERMS MADE CHILD-FRIENDLY

Words that imply pain are naturally fear provoking for children, as well as for adults. Words such as "needles," "shots," "drills," "pulling teeth," and "blood" understandably provoke anxiety and a desire to escape. Since the dentist can now virtually guarantee to control or at least minimize any pain related to procedures (see below), the use of euphemistic and child-oriented terms is morally acceptable and helpful. Using such terms is not lying to or tricking children. It is not like giving a child an intramuscular injection, for example, and saying that "this is just a little mosquito bite—it won't hurt." Children don't easily forgive or forget such betrayals.

Dental schools teach students the importance of being truthful with children about a sensation they will experience but avoiding emotive and anxiety-provoking words. Dentists have success in curtailing the child's fears, first, because they generally manage to prevent or minimize the occurrence of pain, and second, because they use everyday language from the child's point of view. While talking to younger children in a friendly, chatty manner, they use everyday words to describe the equipment that the child may see and the sensations that the child will experience. The young child then knows what to expect. Here are some popular terms:

- The explorer may be called a tooth counter, tooth tickler, or pointer.
- The hand piece used for cleaning teeth is often called the electric toothbrush.
- X-rays are usually called pictures of your teeth or special pictures.
- Local anesthetic is often called sleepy water, magic water, or sleepy medicine.
- The injection of anesthetic may be referred to as a sting, push, pinch, or squirt to put the tooth to sleep.
- The rubber dam may called a raincoat, rubber mask, or tooth raincoat.

- The drill may be called Mr. Whistle, tooth washer, sugarbug chaser, or buzzer.
- The suction may be called Mr. Thirsty.
- Extracting a tooth is called helping your tooth out or wiggling your tooth out.

It is best, therefore, to give the dentist or another member of the dental team the opportunity to describe in their words what will happen. It will usually be much less fear-provoking for your child. You may also use some of these terms at home or when you're coming for your next appointment.

TODDLERS

At this age children do not like being separated from their parents. For children aged one to three, the dentist usually examines a child in what is called the lap-to-lap technique, in which the parent sits knee to knee with the dentist. The parent holds the child on his or her lap, with the child's head on the dentist's knees. The dentist can then carefully check the child's teeth and gums for any signs of infection, the beginnings of decay, or evidence of injury. This takes only a few minutes, and the position also allows the parent a good view. Provided that nothing untoward is found in the examination, the dentist and parent usually discuss home care and preventive strategies. This includes how to brush the child's teeth and caution on the use of the bottle, especially at night.

CHILDREN AGED THREE TO TEN YEARS

Children at this age are able to sit by themselves in the dental chair, with or without their parent's help. Dentists rely on team work to successfully treat children. The dental assistant usually explains the set-up and equipment. The session may start with the assistant asking the child to open her mouth wide so that she can have a "look-see" and to count the teeth that have gone or the teeth that are coming. The child is told what to do to help, such as holding the suction (Mr. Thirsty) to take the saliva away or watching carefully in the hand-held mirror. The assistant also explains what the child should do if anything is bothersome. The commonly accepted "stop" signal is to raise a hand; at this signal the team will stop. In this way the child is incorporated into the team as a "helper."

References to what help the child has given should be voiced spontaneously as part of a successful visit for this age group. Comments such as "You sat so still" or "I know it was uncomfortable holding your mouth open so wide, but I sure got a good look at those molars coming in!" are a helpful guide to children. Making the range of dental experiences normal for children in this age group happens in small and progressive steps. Regular (approximately every six months) preventive dental visits really help to develop positive dental attitudes as well as the brushing and flossing skills needed to prevent dental decay and pain.

From a preschool- or school-aged child's point of view, one of the easiest ways to learn about dentistry is to watch another child, preferably a sibling or friend, having his teeth checked, cleaned, and counted. Seeing another child coping by sitting in the chair, with an open mouth, relatively still and comfortable for a short time, is highly reassuring. Young children learn very rapidly through observing, imitating, and modeling. They tend to have more trust that a situation is inherently safe when this information is obtained from another child than when it is obtained from an adult saying, "It'll be fine."

Observational learning or modeling can, however, account for some of the fears children pick up about going to the dentist. These can be learned from other children, siblings, friends, or parents who have had negative experiences in the dental office. Ensure that the models for your child about coping at the dentist's are positive, helpful ones. If your child inadvertently hears some scary stories, be sure to place them in context, drawing clear distinctions between those stories and your child's situation.

OLDER CHILDREN AND TEENAGERS

Generally by their teen years, adolescents will have had some dental experiences—for better or for worse—but will know what to expect. If a child or teen has had some negative experiences with a particular dentist, it is always a good idea to review the situation, preferably with your child, and decide whether you want to stay with that dentist or go to another. It is very important that the child or adolescent feel good about her dentist. Even if the procedure, such as orthodontic work, is not the most pleasant, if the relationship with the dentist is good, the child will feel respected, supported, and helped.

When an older child is feeling fearful, the child may regress and revert to behavior typical of younger children. Therefore, frightened older children may want their parents present. They may be restless in the chair and wriggle. They could protest or cry at the earliest sign of discomfort. This is when the skills of the team will be put to the test. Can they regain the child's or teen's trust? Will they give the child some control, allow the child to pace the procedure so that it can become more tolerable, and give the child choices? Will they do this in a respectful way so that the child or teen doesn't feel belittled? Could they transform this scary experience into an opportunity to cope, to learn and to feel good about it when it is all over—rather than something to feel bad about, and not want to continue or return?

CHILDREN WHO ARE CHALLENGED

The dentist and the dental team rely on and particularly value the parents of children who are physically, intellectually, or emotionally challenged. These parents provide crucial guidance during dental treatment, particularly during the child's first dental visit or first visit in a new setting. For example, in an open-plan pediatric dental office, if the child is slow to "warm up" to new situations, it is often helpful to sit on a bench with your child, watching other children come and go to have their teeth cleaned. This provides opportunities for the child to explore, play with toys, and assimilate the environment in a non-stressful way. For newcomers in general, there are some advantages to being kept waiting for a first appointment. It allows you to observe, settle in, and become relaxed and oriented.

Many pediatric dental offices have a quiet room for children who are disruptive and noisy or who may upset other children in the office. The most common use of this room is for the examination of young children who, very commonly, cry very noisily when having their teeth examined even when being held by a parent. Being treated in the quiet room, however, may not always be in the best interests of the child. Dr. Penny Leggott was treating a severely autistic 11-year-old child, who tended to be very disruptive, noisy, and combative. He was generally seen for his recall examinations in the quiet room with his mother and father present. On one occasion, the quiet room was in use, so Sam was seated in a chair in the open area, where he could see three other children seated around him. Much to everyone's surprise, including his mother's, instead of protesting, he was much more cooperative than usual and was relatively quiet. Afterward, his mother said that she had begun to realize that Sam was sensitive to peer pressure and that this had clearly operated at the dentist's office. Her story is a reminder that children are continually growing, changing individuals and that we need to remain flexible whatever the child's temperament or restrictions. It also reminds us to provide new opportunities for children as the occasion arises and not to be held back by our assumptions about the child's previous ability and capacity.

Creating a Child-Oriented Environment

Some dental offices, particularly those specializing in children, make the office a playful environment. Some include video monitors so that the child can watch a video while sitting in the dental chair, dress-up clothes, toys, and other child-oriented experiences. Although children enjoy these "extras," they aren't essential for a successful visit to the dentist.

The majority of children are successfully treated in general dental offices that have no special modifications. Having a pleasant environment with interesting pictures on the walls, mobiles, and books will establish a comfortable atmosphere for many children. But going to a pediatric dental office, where the design of the office is entirely child-oriented, can be very reassuring, especially for younger children and toddlers. It also provides the opportunity for children to observe other children undergoing a variety of dental procedures and helps them become accustomed to dental experiences much more quickly. Allowing children to choose a reward, however small, at the end of their procedure is another common practice in child-oriented offices. Receiving a reward enables the child to leave the office with a sense of success, however trying the session.

WHEN A CHILD IS IN PAIN

If a child has not been to the dentist's office before and has been brought in because of dental pain or injury, he will understandably be frightened and tense and may regress behaviorally. Pain is unsettling. The child is uncertain about what will happen—and often the parent is too. Allow your child to revert to comforting, earlier ways of behaving if that helps him. It is the dental team's responsibility to help a child settle and cope with the dental visit.

Let the dental staff take over and make your child feel comfortable. They are trained to do this and can be called upon to do it again. In fact, they need to establish a working alliance and some degree of trust and cooperation for the work to proceed. A parent's support and understanding are key elements. Some older children may also benefit from having a parent present, whereas other children do better when their parents are not present. Staff should be able to support a child's coping in a taxing situation of pain and distress.

This 11-year-old chose to be on her own and spontaneously drew on a distraction method. She tells how she diverted her attention to a more pleasant alternative:

Our dentist has this music, see, and I say to him turn it up real loud. Then I pretend that I have to really learn the music, like the tune, or something terrible will happen to me. And I keep telling myself to listen, listen, listen, and after a while sometimes I almost don't know I'm getting drilled. (Ross and Ross, p. 54)

HOW PAIN IS CONTROLLED IN THE DENTIST'S OFFICE

Pre-emptive and well-planned pain management practices are transforming dental experiences for children. Even invasive procedures such as fillings and extractions need no longer be painful. To prevent pain during these procedures dentists commonly first use a topical anesthetic cream, which comes in a variety of child-friendly flavors, including bubble gum, banana, cherry, and mint. The cream takes approximately one minute to anesthetize the gum. Then the local anesthetic is injected into the anesthetized gum to numb the tooth.

The discomfort caused by injecting a local anesthetic can be controlled by slowly and carefully injecting the solution. In addition, creating distracting sensations by wiggling the cheek help minimize or change the uncomfortable and painful sensations into "tingles." A careful injection technique usually ensures that the child is largely unaware of pain as the local anesthetic infiltrates into the gum. All the child may feel is some of the tingly "weird" feelings as the tooth is going to sleep. The local anesthesia takes effect quite rapidly, within about three to five minutes. Anesthesia in children is usually very easily accomplished.

Very young children may become distressed at the feeling of a "frozen" face. Parent's repeated explanations that the "nerves are still sleeping" may help the child tolerate the strange feeling without being frightened. The effect of a numb face lasts long after the conclusion of the dental visit, taking two to three hours to wear off, after which time the feelings in the child's face gradually return to normal.

Orthodontics

Orthodontics is the one area of dentistry for children that is not pain-free. Children report that orthodontic procedures are painful, and the most painful procedures are the first fitting of the braces and the periodic adjustments, particularly the tightening of the braces. Some children report discomfort between treatments as well. If children are well prepared for orthodontic procedures by the staff, they are more likely to remain committed to their treatments and to continue them, however painful.

Involving children in the decision to start the treatment and giving them a choice to stop if they wish greatly contributes to their capacity to weather the treatments and endure the discomfort and pain. Mild analgesics, such as acetaminophen, are generally used to relieve orthodontic-related pain, which is also lessened when children eat soft foods, such as soup and ice cream, and maintain good dental hygiene following a procedure.

Common Dental Problems and Their Solutions

For some children who have had a negative experience in the dental chair, skilled and sympathetic work by the dental team can mitigate the effects of this experience in the subsequent visit. Other children, however, particularly those who are more sensitive or cautious, have a harder time recovering from the shock of pain in the dentist chair. For these children, one bad experience can destroy their trust and feeling of safety when they are at the dentist's.

Some of the common reasons children may develop anxiety about visiting the dentist include unexpected pain, inadequate preparation for an uncomfortable procedure, major dental work that causes pain and distress, an active gag reflex, or the non-supportive manner of the dentist. How to handle some of these problems is discussed below. If not addressed either by parents or by a professional skilled in handling children's anxieties, these fears can become phobias.

UNEXPECTED PAIN

Even with the best precautions, occasionally local anesthesia is not adequate or a child may perceive pressure or noise as discomfort or pain, especially if the child is very anxious. The dentist should immediately and carefully assess the situation, explain what is going on, reassure the child, and re-anesthetize the child if appropriate. All these steps can help maintain or rebuild confidence.

DENTIST WHO LACKS PATIENCE AND EMPATHY

Not all dentists like treating children. The best solution is to find someone who does.

EXCESSIVE FEARS

A few children develop excessive fears over time. This dental phobia can be so great that it is almost impossible for them to undergo routine dental care without help. A dentist who is skilled in communication and has a good staff may be able to manage these children with the help of nitrous oxide (a quick-acting and relatively safe gas, also known as laughing gas), local anesthesia, and a caring and empathetic manner. Some children, however, may need additional help, such as psychotherapy or hypnosis, to control their anxiety.

Case Study: Not all situations go smoothly

Six-year-old red-haired Theo had numerous cavities because his teeth naturally had very thin enamel. After X-rays and a careful examination, his dentist said Theo would need to have four or perhaps five fillings done quite promptly. Theo, an intelligent and thoughtful boy, was overwhelmed by the news. The dental team began the procedure by giving Theo local anesthetic and then putting a rubber dam* in his mouth. This new, uncomfortable experience unsettled Theo, who began whimpering and wriggling. The dentist said in a kindly way: "It is important that we carry on, because we will have at least another two or three more visits to get all your teeth fixed." This statement unsettled Theo even more. He tensed up and said, "I don't want that thing in my mouth!" The dentist then said he couldn't do this extensive work without the dam, and maybe they should consider doing the whole procedure under general anesthetic. Theo's mother went white. "No!" she said. "Let's think about what else could help Theo." The dentist then suggested they look into some help for Theo and ended the session.

Less than happy, Theo's mother took Theo for psychotherapy geared specifically toward enabling him to cope with the dental procedures. It turned out that what troubled Theo the most was "having that thing across my throat." It became apparent that if the dam were eliminated Theo could handle the fillings using some coping methods. In the following two psychotherapy sessions, Theo learned and practiced relaxation and imagery methods recorded onto audio-tapes. Lying on a reclining chair, relaxing his mouth wide open, he focused on this tape in his own Walkman, newly acquired for the purpose. The tapes took him hang-gliding through the Grand Canyon, down through the different sedimentary levels so that he could study all the different ages embedded in the rocks. He gradually sailed down to the powerful Colorado River below, where he transferred onto a river raft.

---

* The rubber dam helps protect the child from accidentally swallowing or breathing in old fillings, or decayed tooth material during dental work. Many dentists cut a "breathing hole" in the dam, and the majority of children are comfortable with the dam.

Theo's motivation was impressive. A consultation was set up between his psychotherapist, his mother, and the dentist to determine if he were prepared to do the procedures without a dam. The difference was that this time Theo was highly motivated, informed, prepared, and relaxed, and he would be hang-gliding in his mind. The answer was yes, and to his mother's relief Theo went on to complete all of his treatment with a tremendous feeling of accomplishment.

GAGGING

Many children have an active gag reflex that gradually diminishes as they get older. When a child becomes anxious and scared that she may gag during dental work, it inevitably occurs more frequently. There are a number of techniques that can help:

- Partially sitting up instead of fully reclining in the dental chair can diminish the likelihood of gagging.
- Nitrous oxide can help reduce the gag reflex.
- Topical anesthetic sprayed on the back of the tongue and palate helps.
- Gaining the child's confidence and taking the procedures in small steps is useful.
- Using hypnosis or diverting attention often works.

Case Study: Jeremy's triumph

Fourteen-year-old Jeremy had a long history of dental fears—no awful experiences that he can recall, but the fear was always there. He says that it faded a lot when he was around nine years old, but an automatic gagging reflex remained whenever the dentist put an instrument into the back of his mouth or touched his sensitive tongue. This is what Jeremy wrote in an essay on his experience:

I did not want to gag. I tried really hard not to, but it was like a conditioned reflex. When I would gag it felt like I couldn't breathe. I would be out of breath and feel very nauseous. My eyes would water too. Even though the gag would only last a second, it seemed like a lot longer. It was very scary.

I went to the dentist. I had eight teeth that needed to be sealed. All of them were at the back of my mouth. One is bad enough, and I could probably have handled it, but there were eight! My dentist was very supportive that I try hypnosis. So Dr. K. taught me breathing techniques and then together over some months we worked on a number of different suggestions, strategies, and hypnosis tapes to overcome my problem. On the tapes were messages about how I could keep my mouth open without gagging.

Night after night I would listen to these tapes as I fell asleep. My family was very supportive. I practiced seeing how many teaspoons I could get into my mouth. I could get three pretty far back without gagging. There I was, walking around my house with my mouth wide open and spoons sticking out. It turned into a habit. Once I even walked in on my mom when she had a friend over, with my spoons sticking out of my mouth. The hypnosis was working.

Dr. K spoke to my dentist on a number of occasions. He was very supportive. They went over the procedure; all my teeth were not going to be done at the same time. The job would be completed over a number of appointments. There were going to be no needles, and no pain. That was the relieving news, but I was still a little nervous. My first appointment was in September. I had major butterflies that day and the night before. I used one of the tapes. But to my surprise I did well. A lot better than I thought I'd do. There was almost no gagging, but I was still not satisfied. I wanted NO GAGGING! Call me stubborn, but if you're going to do something, do it right!

I should mention this is no individual effort. We worked as a team, my dentist, Dr. K, and me. We took the problem, and if there were still some kinks, we improved on them. That's why we went through four tapes; we kept getting new ideas. Knowing all of that comforted me on my second visit. In a sense it was not just me in the chair but Dr. K was there too. Not her, but her voice, which was coming out of my Walkman.

After my second appointment I was so happy. I had accomplished what I had set out to do. For over half an hour I sat in that chair, my mouth open while my dentist worked on me. And for over half an hour, there was no gagging whatsoever! The dentist also gave me breaks every little while; that helped a lot too. I was on top of the world. I did it! I conquered my problem. I was not the only one who was excited, my family, my dentist, the nurse, Dr. K. They were all proud of me. It felt good.

There is probably no greater feeling than being proud of yourself. I was on cloud nine that whole day. What I'm trying to say is that no matter what, anything can be accomplished. I'm living proof. It's mind over matter. The mind has a lot of power. Being hypnotized was one of the most amazing experiences of my life. What's more amazing is what can be done with it. The mind is a terrible thing to waste!

GENERAL ANESTHESIA FOR MAJOR DENTAL WORK

Most parents fear general anesthesia for their child. Indeed, general anesthesia should not be undertaken lightly. It does, however, provide a means for taking care of extensive dental work for some children under some circumstances—for example, a child under three years old who is too young to understand and cooperate in the dental office but who has extensive decay resulting from use of a night-time bottle of juice; an older, mentally challenged child with numerous cavities; or a child who has extensive dental needs and such extreme anxiety that psychotherapy and behavioral strategies in the office do not work.

SEDATION AND ITS RISKS

It is also a serious matter to use sedation with children in the dental office, and the risks of sedation are not always fully appreciated. Although some people believe that sedation has less serious consequences than anesthesia, this is not necessarily so. It is now established that sedation techniques for young children are generally less reliable than for adults; children can become over excited instead of sedated. The dosage levels often tend to be low to ensure the safety of the child, but this in turn reduces the "sedative" effect. In addition, dentists have noted that many children have negative feelings about dentistry after a series of visits using sedation.

A number of pediatric dentists believe that if all other methods of help and intervention are not effective, general anesthesia may be a better option for extensive work than the use of sedation. Dr. Leggott has observed a number of these children, who, after treatment under general anesthesia in a caring environment such as a children's hospital, return to the dental office for their post-operative visit as cheerful, cooperative, and relaxed young patients. It is clear that even at a very young age, children understand when they have a problem and also understand when the problem has been taken care of. If you find it exasperating sitting through an hour of restorative work at the dentist, imagine how much more difficult it is for your three- or four-year-old to sit through a number of visits if he has extensive dental needs. In these extreme circumstances, treatment under general anesthesia may sometimes be the kindest option for a child's emotional and physical well-being.

Dental Emergencies

There are five steps in handling a dental emergency:

1. Keep calm—as in all emergencies.
2. Take quick action (specifics are below).
3. Explain to your child what you are doing and how it will help.
4. Use acetaminophen if the child is in pain.
5. If the pain persists, see the dentist.

TOOTHACHE

Reassure your child as you clean the area of the painful tooth thoroughly and gently. Rinse your child's mouth vigorously with warm water, and if it is not painful use dental floss to dislodge any impacted food or debris between the teeth. Don't place aspirin on the aching tooth or gum, since aspirin burns. The child could be given acetaminophen for the pain. If the child's face is swollen, apply a cold compress and see a dentist immediately.

BROKEN TOOTH

Reassure the child, adding that you can help. Rinse the injured area with *warm* water. Place a cold compress over the face and the area of the injury to reduce swelling. Locate the tooth, saving any broken tooth fragments, and call for immediate dental help.

BLEEDING AFTER BABY TOOTH FALLS OUT

In general this isn't painful, because the root has resorbed (dissolved) and the remaining "crown" is attached by the gum alone. Fold and pack a clean wet gauze over the bleeding area (if the gauze is wet, it will not pull the blood clot off when it is taken off). Ask your child to bite on the gauze with pressure for up to 15 minutes. Congratulate your child. Remind her that the tooth fairy will visit, and be sure to place a reward under her pillow. If bleeding recurs, repeat biting down on the wet gauze for another 15 minutes. If it doesn't settle, see a dentist.

KNOCKED-OUT PERMANENT TOOTH

Find the tooth and hold it by the crown, *not* by the root. You may carefully rinse the tooth, but don't handle it unnecessarily. Reassure the child that you may be able to save the tooth. Inspect the tooth for fractures. If it is sound, try to reinsert it in its socket. Press down on the tooth gently until the biting edge is level with the adjacent tooth, or with the same tooth on the other side. Have the child stabilize the tooth in place by biting on a piece of gauze.

If you cannot reinsert the tooth, carry it in a cup containing the child's saliva or cold water. The tooth may also be carried in the child's mouth, tucked into her cheek; there is a risk that the tooth may be swallowed, however, so be careful. Time is a critical factor in saving the tooth so see a dentist immediately. If replaced within 15 minutes, the tooth may do well. If there is a two-hour delay, it is unlikely that the tooth can be saved. (A tetanus booster injection may be needed after the reinsertion of a tooth.)

CUT OR BITTEN TONGUE, LIP, OR CHEEK

Tell your child that he is lucky that he bit his lip or the inside of his cheek, because this part heals much more quickly than the outside. Apply ice to the bruised area, or have your child suck a popsicle or ice chips. Usually this pain stings sharply at first and subsides quite rapidly, particularly with cold or ice. If there is bleeding, apply gentle pressure with a piece of gauze or cloth. If the bleeding does not stop after 15 minutes or cannot be controlled by simple pressure, take the child to the hospital. Keeping teeth clean and rinsing three or four times a day with water or an oral liquid rinse will help prevent infection and speed healing.

COLD OR CANKER SORES

Mouth ulcers or canker sores are painful shallow white sores in the lining of the mouth, the gums, or the inside of the lips or cheek, and they can be a recurring problem for some children. For healing and pain relief, ask the child to swish a solution made up of a half teaspoon of sodium bicarbonate (baking soda) in a cup of warm water for a minute after eating. Acetaminophen may be helpful if pain persists. In addition, commercially available local anesthetic gel or cream can be placed on the ulcer before eating to temporarily numb the area and make eating more comfortable. Tooth brushing may be painful until the sore heals, so use careful brushing that avoids the ulcer.

Conclusion

To ensure a positive experience at the dentist's office, make regular appointments with the same dentist. Over time, as the child grows and matures, she will learn what to expect, and how to participate in making the dental visit a pleasant experience. These visits should reflect flexibility and attentiveness to the developmental and individual needs of each child. These characteristics are fundamental to any good health care program and also help establish a regular working alliance, a good relationship, and a feeling of safety and trust between health care provider and patient.

Since the child's fear of pain may be even more of a problem than the occurrence of pain itself during dental procedures, creating a positive attitude toward dental work through successive good experiences visiting the dentist makes children less fearful. In the main, pain in pediatric dentistry is preventable; and if it does occur, the pain can be quickly controlled. In many respects, the management of pain and anxiety in dentistry is a model for other areas of health care.

CHAPTER 11

Emergency Pain In Hospital

FEW EXPERIENCES ARE AS UNSETTLING to both parents and child as the treatment for pain in hospital, whether this is an anticipated treatment or an emergency treatment. Nevertheless, if parents are prepared and have prepared their child, the uncertainties and apprehensions can be minimized and the experience can be made manageable.

Preparing for Emergencies

"Emergencies are hard because they take you by surprise!" says a daycare organizer at a downtown toddler-infant facility. Taking care of over 80 young children, she knows the problem from experience. She adds that because you never really have an opportunity for practice, it is important to have all the information you need and a well-established emergency routine. The emergency routine established at that daycare begins with a call to the child's parents, followed by a call to the pediatrician. The parents are then called again so that a meeting place, such as the emergency room or the doctor's office, can be arranged.

Now is the time to think about what you, as a parent or a professional working with children, would do in an emergency:

- Whom do you call first?
- How do you assess the child's condition?
- How have you responded in previous crises, emergencies, or accidents?
- Do you remember how you felt, what helped, and what didn't?
- Did you experience a sense of helplessness?
- Have you taken a first-aid course that includes CPR? The value of a first-aid course, which often involves only one day of training, cannot be overestimated. You learn the ABCs of life-saving actions, designed to effectively assess and aid someone in the midst of physical trauma.

Forced to depend on the opinions of others in an emergency, you are thrust into a new relationship with your child and the medical caretakers. Once again, however, your role is pivotal as you explain and interpret to the child what is happening and what will happen.

When choosing an emergency facility, it is crucial to ensure that the facility is equipped for pediatric emergencies, that it has personnel trained to treat children and equipment designed for children's smaller bodies. Because they have smaller lungs and airways, children are at greater risk for breathing problems than adults and require plastic airway tubes less than half the width of those made for adults. Similarly, doses of analgesics and other medication must be adjusted for the child's smaller body. Therefore, it is wise to discuss with your physician what facility you should take your child to in an emergency. Note, however, that in a life-threatening emergency the ambulance will go to the closest hospital.

Experiencing Emergencies

During an emergency, take the following steps:

- Stay as calm as possible; this is the key to coping.
- Call 911.
- Determine who is in charge in the emergency situation.
- Carry out life-saving measures, such as CPR.
- Keep the child warm until the ambulance or doctor arrives.
- Acknowledge the facts of the situation and reassure the child that help is on the way and that soon things will get better. Believe that what you are saying is true—while believing too in the resiliency of children and their ability to be helped. You could say: "Did you know your brain and body are very smart at working together? They are—and they are already doing that. That's why they are sending you that signal of hurting so you can know and can tell us, and that helps us to know how to help you. So you can rest and let yourself relax so that your brain and body can work inside of you to start healing now."
- In an emergency dash with your child to hospital, the time you have to prepare your child for what awaits starts from the moment of the accident: "Oh goodness! You have a cut. It's hurting a lot and it will stop. Yes, it is bleeding and that will stop too, so we'll put this clean wet gauze on and wrap it carefully to help the blood to stop and clot. Your blood knows how to do that well. I think we're going to take care of this immediately— we're off to the hospital so that the cut can be checked out and will be sure to heal quickly."

If there is time, bring along the following:

- The child's medical insurance card and hospital card, if available;
- A container of any medication she is taking;
- Any items that can explain the injury or pain, such as toxic materials;
- A change of clothing; and
- A favorite blanket or toy and books.

Case Study: My dash to the hospital

I put the banana cake into the 350-degree oven, closed the oven door, and turned around to wash the utensils. In a two-second flash, curious 14-month-old Daniel pulled open the oven door and put his chubby right hand onto the burning hot rack! It happened so rapidly I was stunned. Almost reflexively I swiftly lifted him, and immediately ran cold water over his hand while yelling for help. My husband came and called our close friend Jo, who fortunately worked as an occupational therapist in the local burn unit. He then called the hospital to alert them that we were on our way. Jo drove us to emergency with a bag of frozen peas wrapped in a towel around Daniel's burned hand. Through Daniel's frantic crying I held him, telling him, "Let the peas take some of the hot owie away, feel how nice and cold it is . . . the heat was for the cake, not your hand. Your hand can now get cold, Daniel, cold, cold like snow, cold snow. We'll soon be at the hospital; they'll have powerful medicine to take all the pain away." I attempted to soothe and comfort the confused and distressed little guy on a ride that seemed endless.

Carrying Daniel through the doors of emergency I heard my voice yell out, "It's burns!"* A nurse promptly gave him an injection of codeine. Flamazine and bandages were ready, and within less than a minute after the codeine, Daniel was deeply asleep. It was then easy to examine his hand to determine that although all four fingers had experienced second- and third-degree burns, the wounds were not so extensive that the skin wouldn't knit together. The prognosis looked good. I just had to get him used to the routine of daily hand-soaks in warm water and bandage changes, made easier with his favorite songs. Since then Daniel has had no fears about returning to hospital, which he has had to do more times than I wanted. Being vigorous exacts a price, but practice at least has its benefits! Daniel's repertoire for managing pain and anxiety includes blowing, rubbing, talking to himself, and singing.

---

*Hearing one's voice in a disembodied way is a form of dissociation (discussed in the section on hypnosis in chapter 6) commonly experienced when one is in shock. All my attention was on Daniel, and my reactions appeared not to belong to me.

IN THE AMBULANCE

As you travel in the ambulance, say what you can be sure is on the child's mind: that you know she hurts, is afraid. Reframe her thoughts to *undo the uncertainty*. Comments from well-meaning professionals (the ambulance driver, paramedics, emergency room receptionists, and nurses and doctors) such as "I'm not sure what's happening here . . ." can inadvertently contribute to uncertainty. You can reframe the scary situation of driving in the ambulance by saying: "I'm glad that we're in the ambulance now, and you'll probably be surprised how fast we'll get there. It's pretty interesting here." Reminding the child that you are there and "in touch" will serve as a strong source of comfort both en route and after arrival.

Provide the child with some information about what will happen once you arrive at the hospital, such as, "We'll probably meet a bunch of new people asking a lot of questions. You can remember their names if you want—I'll help—but be sure to tell them exactly how you are feeling, what hurts, and what doesn't so they'll know how to help best." For the child who is afraid or overwhelmed at the prospect of talking to strangers, prompt him to let them know: "It's hard for me to talk now," or, if talking increases his distress, he could say: "It hurts more when I talk." You may wish to ask the child the questions to which you need answers to ensure that you understand and can therefore accurately represent the problems, worries, and discomfort to the doctor. Knowing that you are there to serve as an anchor and to represent the child's needs is a great reassurance to an overwhelmed child in pain.

IN THE EMERGENCY ROOM

Preparation, explanation, orientation, and mobilization of your child's coping skills continue upon your arrival at the emergency room, during treatment, and after the treatment is completed. All of these steps may take longer than you wish, so use the time well:

- Talk to your child even if she seems unconscious. Your voice is deeply and intimately familiar and will convey your continuing contact and love.
- Tell your child exactly what is happening so that he can settle back into resting and not fighting or being frightened.
- Remind your child that her body can do what it needs to get well right now.

- Keep physical contact by holding or stroking a non-painful area of the child's body to comfort and reassure him and to provide a competing, pleasant sensation.
- Be sure to relate important medical information to the team on your arrival, such as whether your child has diabetes or asthma or is allergic to a particular medication. Ensure that the physician who attends your child also has this information.
- If you sense that a decision may not be the best for your child, be sure to tell the physician. Here is one instance: "I'm worried about your giving my child penicillin, because I am allergic to it, as is my aunt. I would hate her to have an allergic reaction to the medication on top of her fever and pain."
- Stay with your child in the emergency room and let the staff know that you can and will be of help. Continue to talk to your child, explaining any of the puzzling sounds, sights, or procedures in the emergency room. Be sure to explain and minimize other children's cries of distress, since these can otherwise negatively affect an unsure or frightened child.
- Request pain medication if you know that your child is in pain; sometimes a child's cry can be interpreted by hospital staff as an expression of fear instead of pain and fear.

Frequently in the emergency department, where quick and correct decisions about medical interventions need to be made, parents can play a pivotal role in ensuring that these decisions are in the best interests of the child. The following case study shows why medical and nursing staff should trust parents' judgment or intuition and the problems that can arise if they don't.

Case Study: A parent's intuition

Four-year-old Silas had been complaining of a sore tummy for two days. On the third day he was fine in the morning, but that afternoon he screamed with sudden pain that was like long cramps and then lay on the coach, whimpering on and off with pain.

Sensing that something more serious was occurring, his mother took him to the nearest emergency room, where they waited for at least an hour (it was crowded) before a physician briefly questioned and examined Silas. In passing, Silas's mother said to the physician, "He often gets these stomach aches, sometimes even once a week, but this time it seems worse and a little different, sort of like cramps." The physician responded, "You know abdominal pain like this is very common in young children like Silas (by now Silas was a bit perkier and almost smiling). It doesn't seem to be very serious. I don't think it's his appendix, and he hasn't had any diarrhea, has he?" "No," said his mother, "but even though he looks a bit better right now he was in quite a bit of pain just a little while ago." "Well," said the physician, "I'll give you a prescription for Tylenol #3, which is a strong pain medication and has codeine in it. But I suggest you watch him, and if his stomach doesn't settle, bring him back."

Silas's mother didn't feel happy about the decision; she had a sixth sense that something else was going on, but the emergency room was so busy, the staff seemed so stretched, and Silas seemed to be a bit better. So she bought the medication from the pharmacist on the way home and gave Silas his first dose. Within the hour he was asleep, but when he awakened a few hours later, he was screaming and writhing, doubled over in pain. She gave Silas another dose of medication before putting him into her car and dashing to the nearest emergency room.

Carrying Silas into the case room, she said in a strong voice that surprised her: "My son is in a lot of pain—there is something very wrong with his bowel or stomach or something. Please help!" The emergency room staff immediately took Silas to a cubicle. After reviewing the history with his mother and carefully examining Silas, the physician said that clearly this was not "just another sore tummy." He suspected that it might be a kind of bowel obstruction called an intussusception, and he explained that a special X-ray would tell whether that was the problem. If so, an X-ray procedure with barium might be the right treatment, and surgery might be avoided. The intussusception was confirmed and corrected—the obstruction was relieved by the X-ray and Silas was able to go home the same day. It turns out that the codeine medication in the prescription Tylenol prescribed to take the pain away also slowed the normal movement of the bowels, making the partial obstruction worse.

Afterward, on reflection, Silas's mother remarked that she knew she had not conveyed enough key facts that would have made the physician take a more considered look at her child's pain and suspect something more serious. For his part, the physician probably had not asked enough questions about the nature of Silas' pain. If he had inquired and found out about the sudden painful cramping Silas had experienced, the physician's suspicions might have increased. But he didn't know Silas. His mother knew that Silas's behavior was out of character for him, but in the busy emergency room it must have looked mild. Through this experience Silas's mother learned not only to trust her intuition but also to make sure that as Silas's best advocate she express her sixth sense and give all the details of her child's pain, even when she is not asked directly.

COMMUNICATING WITH NURSES AND PHYSICIANS

In advocating for your child, be sure to accurately represent his views to the doctor. If the child can do something for himself, then the parent may wish to make sure that happens by saying directly to the nurse or doctor, "Jimmy would like to talk with you about how he's feeling and what you're going to do next before you go on. Could you do this please?" You may need to "monitor" what the doctor says, as it is being said, so that you can modify any "scary" words that he or she may inadvertently use.

CONVEYING INFORMATION WITH A FUTURE ORIENTATION

To minimize anxiety and uncertainty, attempt to get information about your child's condition or treatments as early as possible so that you can relay it to the child, if the staff has not yet done so. "Will we be going home after the stitches? ("after a cast is put on?" "after a test is done and medication prescribed?") If you are going home, talk with the child about what you will do there, how proud you are of her cooperation, to whom she will tell her story. Or, if it is certain that the child will be admitted to the hospital, tell her that, explaining that the hospital room will be more private than the emergency room, although she may be sharing it with one or more children who have pain or who are also ill. But it will be calmer, with less hullabaloo, and she will continue to have all the support and care she needs to get well.

PAIN MANAGEMENT IN THE EMERGENCY ROOM

Children's pain in the emergency room is quite often acute pain. For a traumatic injury or other painful medical condition, acute pain serves a protective and useful purpose, warning the child that tissue damage has occurred and that he should avoid moving or using that part of the body. Feeling for the pain in the child's body, however, may itself be painful, temporarily causing more pain in a child who already feels uncomfortable. A child's acute pain thus also helps the emergency physician to identify where the injury or infection is occurring and, together with other symptoms, leads to a diagnosis. For example, acute pain in the right lower abdomen, together with symptoms of a fever and perhaps vomiting, may often (but not always) lead to a diagnosis of acute appendicitis.

If the child experiences more pain and discomfort during the physical examination, the adult accompanying the child can encourage the child to "blow away the pain," to focus on an interesting poster, or to count the buttons on your sweater as a coping distraction during this necessary but painful examination. (The fact that the child is distracted and is not as bothered by the pain does not mean that the pain is not there, but that she is coping better with it than before.) Physicians should explain what they are doing before and during the examination to minimize any potential discomfort.

The adult accompanying the distressed child needs to ensure that the child in pain is given analgesic medication and experiences adequate relief. Studies of pain practices in emergency rooms suggest that there is still some reluctance to give the more powerful pain medications, such as morphine, to younger children in severe pain. Unfounded fears of addiction or respiratory depression, unlikely to occur with the appropriate doses, are still prevalent. If, however, a diagnosis is difficult to reach for a disease or trauma, the staff may hold off for a while before providing an opioid, since the symptoms, although distressing, need to be carefully followed to establish a diagnosis. When a child in the emergency room experiences high-intensity pain whose origin is known, such as from burns, a fractured limb, or sickle cell disease, whatever the age of the child, morphine or opioid medication (see p. 182) is the standard method of pain relief.

In the emergency room, because of the urgent nature of the pain the child is experiencing, analgesic medications are often given intravenously, through a fine-gauge needle inserted into a vein in the child's hand, arm, or foot. The pain relief is usually almost immediate, and side effects can easily be monitored. Since the local anesthetic cream EMLA® requires a minimum of an hour to become effective as an anesthetic, it may not be useful in time-limited situations in the emergency room. Although needles are never pleasant for children (see pp. 306–312 for ways to coach your child through this), until there are alternative routes of delivering analgesia rapidly to children in pain, the use of needles, as in an IV or an injection, will remain commonplace in the emergency room.

Of all the forms of needles, receiving an intramuscular injection is the most painful. Therefore, if it can be avoided, it should be. Ask the attending physician whether the prescribed medication is available in oral form or whether other medications are going to be given to the child via an IV. If so, ask whether this medication can be added to the IV in order to make it easier on the child and provide a more steady level of analgesic medication.

Local anesthetics are frequently used to numb an area before a wound is sutured. Although most local anesthetics are in injectable form, some topical local anesthetics, such as TAC (tetracaine, adrenaline, and cocaine) can be applied to some wounds before suturing and aid in creating effective anesthesia quickly. Ask if such a topical anesthetic is available and suitable for your child. Since it is child-friendly, it is less likely to cause anxiety and may also increase the child's cooperation.

Hypnosis, imagery, massage, TENS, and many of the other methods outlined in chapter 6 can also be useful in helping a child in pain to cope during emergency room treatment. All of these methods work well in combination with analgesics. In addition to helping the child feel better, these methods increase his sense of self-reliance and trust that he is being helped.

Case Study: Giving a child more time

If there is leeway and a child is clearly overwhelmed and not mentally or emotionally ready to undergo a painful procedure, give the child more time, even though that may be inconvenient. Here is an example:

Seven-year-old Susie, an imaginative, sensitive child, was in a playground accident in which the tip of a pencil broke off and lodged in her cheek. Knowing that the graphite should not remain in her child's skin, her mother immediately took her into the emergency department of their local hospital, thinking that it would have to come out promptly or it might cause an infection. Susie was terrified and refused to allow the physician to remove the graphite using local anesthetic. She said in retrospect: "I wasn't really prepared. It was like he just said, 'I could take it out now!' It was too quick. I wasn't ready . . . I always hate getting my splinters out! I wanted to know what was going to happen, then I could organize myself. If he just took it out, I wouldn't be able to breathe, I wouldn't know what was going to happen, then it would make me really scared. I needed time to get used to the idea and then know what was going to happen."

Fortunately, the physician understood and respected Susie's wishes, and since the wound was minor, he rescheduled her for the procedure a week later. This time Susie was ready. Plans had been made, and instead of relying only on the painful injectable local anesthetic, Susie's mother had obtained EMLA®, *the cream-based local anesthetic, put it on Susie's cheek, and covered it with the special bandage 90 minutes before surgery so that her skin would be anesthetized. Susie said having the extra time, the cream, and her mom's hand to squeeze during the brief surgery to remove the pencil tip helped the most.*

The child in acute pain in the emergency room may find herself in many different places, including admission, the emergency cubicle, X-ray, and the waiting area. In all of these places the child will do best when she knows exactly what is going to happen, when, for how long, why, and by whom. Legitimate expressed or unexpressed concerns in most children's minds might be: "I'm afraid; do I have to do this?" "How long will it take?" "I don't want to move anymore; I hurt more when I move," and "When will it be over?" You must respond to these anxieties, articulating what you think is on the child's mind, assuring her of the need for the process and of people's commitment to do it as safely, properly, quickly, and painlessly as possible. Particularly in the face of the child's (and family's) worry, sadness, helplessness, and pain, reminders that the pain will not last and that relief will come must not be neglected.

IF RESTRAINTS HAVE TO BE USED

At times it is necessary to restrain a child while a wound is being repaired. Trying to stitch a child who is a moving target may cause even more pain than stitching a child who is still. These principles should be followed when using restraint:

- Parents (in the majority of instances) should not be asked or expected to hold the child for a painful procedure.
- Restraints should be used in such a way as to maintain the child's dignity, not in a punitive context or in a manner that leads to feelings of helplessness rather than a measure of self-control.
- If a full-body restraint is to be used, rather than trying to talk the staff out of what seems to be a foregone conclusion beyond your control, describe what is going to happen to the child in this way: "In a few moments the doctor will be ready (to stitch up the cuts/help straighten your leg bone and put on the cast), and so it is very important to be as still as possible. To help you be still, we are going to use this thing that will hold your arms and legs this way [demonstrate]. "One time another boy told me he didn't like this thing at all, so he pretended that he was getting into an astronaut's suit and going to outer space. That way he didn't even think that he was in the room while they were sewing his wound. Or "The girl down the hall was thinking that it was like a costume for a Halloween party. What costume do you want to pretend that it is?" This direct

and natural link to imagery helps the child extract some comfort and control from an otherwise frightening, out-of-control situation.

A child may object, or out of fear say, "That's dumb! It won't help!" Although such reactions may be frustrating, they are neither unusual nor unpredictable. It helps to be ready for some negativity. Responding creatively can go a long way; the support person can continue, "Well, I'm going to pretend that *I'm* an astronaut on Halloween . . ."

After the Emergency Is Over

Going home from the emergency room (or the hospital or the accident scene) is the time to start to make sense of the entire experience. However exhausted or relieved you and your child may feel, sharing your feelings with your child and his with you in the aftermath of an emergency may be as important as, or even more important than, what went on during the experience itself, especially if the experience was traumatic or more negative than you would have liked.

In the immediate aftermath, especially, you have the opportunity— and perhaps even the obligation—to say the right kinds of things in the right way to promote the child's sense of well-being, healing, comfort, and self-confidence. Perhaps most important, use this opportunity to undo any misconceptions of events to prevent them from becoming internalized as fears or negative expectations that could adversely affect how the child experiences and copes with possible future emergencies.

Be alert to negative statements or misperceptions and make an effort to reframe and reshape them in the best interests of your child. If no spontaneous remarks or observations are forthcoming, you might wish to ask something like, "Well, what was the *best thing* about the emergency room?" Such almost ridiculous-sounding comments will certainly get the attention of a child who has just endured some traumatic event. A child may incredulously and angrily say, "Nothing!" This would give you the opportunity to say, "Well, it sounds like the best thing, then, was leaving and finally getting out of there! I'm glad it's over and we're home. I was sure proud of the way you worked with and helped the nurses and doctors."

Since children—and especially young children—often believe that they were responsible for their injury or illness (even if they were not), it is important to let them know that they were not at fault. One easy way of doing so is to compliment and thank them; naming specific ways they helped makes them feel a little better about what occurred. Creating a helpful retrospective becomes particularly important if your child received comments from family or health care workers that he was "acting like a baby" or was "uncooperative."

Having set the tone for discussing the events, you can then ask your child which part she thought was the hardest and help unravel any misconceptions. These could take the form of "Why did the nurse hold me so tight?" or "I hate doctors; it hurt when he put in that needle." Taking the opportunity to discuss such comments will help put some closure on the experience and go a long way toward preventing this experience from becoming generalized into fears or negative responses in the future. You might do this by clarifying: "I'm sure the nurse didn't mean to hurt you or your feelings. She knew that if you held very still, then the (test or stitches) wouldn't bother you as much." Or you can explain again why the local anesthetic was used: "I know that it does sting for awhile when the needle and the numbing medicine go in. The doctor uses it so that the nerves that feel will go to sleep and you won't notice any more hurt—only a little pushing feeling when he puts in the stitches—but that didn't seem to bother you, did it?"

Such simple-sounding explanations are not only appreciated by children but are often pivotal in "wrapping up" the experience in a positive manner. In this way you plant the seed for coping in a helpful way during any future emergencies.

Emergency pain situations can be highly dramatic, and when they are, the experience tends to become imprinted in the minds and memories of family members and the child. However traumatic the experience of emergency pain might be, if thought and effort go into discussing the experience afterward, everyone can come to some degree of resolution and feel that they did the best they could under the circumstances. If not, they learn what could have been more helpful.

CHAPTER 12

Preparation for Hospital

WHEN CHILDREN ARRIVE AT THE HOSPITAL for the first time, it may seem like a strange and bewildering place, with strong, unusual smells and lots of busy, bustling people in a profusion of uniforms. In this setting, the most talkative, independent child can become quiet and clingy. For parents there are different concerns about taking their child into hospital: the worries of a possible illness and its implications, the demands of diagnostic procedures, and the memories of their own previous hospital experiences, among other concerns.

The greatest fear for younger children is being separated from parents; in addition to that anxiety, older children fear pain, discomfort, and surprises. Providing an explanation and discussion of what will happen and what the child can do to help herself is the first step parents can take to make a hospital visit okay. This step is necessary even if the child has been to hospital before. Particularly if a child has had a tough time previously in a medical clinic or hospital, taking the time to ensure that the child feels prepared and supported and has some useful coping strategies will counteract the memories and fears of that previous negative experience.

About Preparation

Unlike emergencies, scheduled surgeries, medical investigations, and medical treatments permit orientation and preparation time. Preparation is a mental, physical, often emotional, and behavioral process. Gathering the necessary information is only one part of becoming prepared; finding out what is involved, feeling a little anxious, attempting to digest your many mixed feelings about what may happen, and even rehearsing how to behave are all important aspects of "becoming ready" to go into hospital.

THE 3 R'S OF PREPARATION

When preparing children for hospital, follow the 3 Rs of preparation—rehearsal, reassurance, and recapitulation.

Rehearsal

In the rehearsal phase, provide the child or teen with the opportunity to know what she will actually experience, not from the medical viewpoint but from her own frame of reference—what she will feel and see, the steps involved in the procedure, and, most important, what coping methods can help make it go well. Then play out or rehearse the procedure with your child.

Reassurance

In the reassurance phase, when the procedure is under way, mitigate any stress by talking calmly and comfortingly about what is happening; encourage using the coping methods; and confirm that your child or teen is handling the situation well. Having some physical contact—such as patting, stroking, or rocking—while you talk is reassuring. If a child does not welcome patting, stroking, or words of reassurance, he may be feeling tired or irritable or may need to cope independently and not to be seen as vulnerable. Accept where your child is and start there; he may not stay there for long.

A *cautionary note:* Since our children read us emotionally with uncanny accuracy, it is important to be genuine. If a situation is very tough, do not provide excessive reassurance or "false cheer," which can make a child feel even more alone and unsupported.

Recapitulation

The final phase, or the aftermath, involves going over what happened, how your preparation worked, what coping methods helped, and, if you had to do it over again, how you would do it next time. This dissecting process—once the heat is off—can be useful as a learning phase and significantly affect future experiences. The benefits can be enormous. Going over what worked and what didn't work also acknowledges your child as the authority on her experience. Recapitulation is a confidence-building experience: no matter how tough the actual hospital encounter was, discussing again what occurred—even a few days or a week later—serves as an opportunity to understand the experience, integrate it into one's life, and gain some mastery over the situation.

PREPARING TO GO TO HOSPITAL

Preparation can also consist of planning details, such as making arrangements for transportation and building a plan with your child that will strengthen your working alliance and, perhaps, your alliance with hospital staff. The multifaceted process of parent and child "gearing up" can effectively promote coping with the strangeness, anxiety, or pain in hospital. Preparation may involve giving the child the opportunity to see the hospital while he is feeling well, to ask questions, to draw pictures, or to describe the details in his journal and to address some fears and uncertainties that occur as he sees the real place. Visiting the hospital also allows your child to begin establishing relationships and some trust in the hospital staff, and to discuss and initiate coping skills.

When a child of any age is actively coping with hospitalization, she is less likely to tangle up the pain with fear of abandonment, white coats, or the unknown. Medical and surgical procedures are intrinsically stressful. With good preparation, those procedures can become manageable, and the pain won't be surprising, terrifying, violating, or overwhelming. Pain is never nice, but it can be made manageable. Extensive research with children going to hospital shows that preparation is a key part of coping better in hospital.

THE IMPORTANCE OF DISCUSSION

Occasionally parents are concerned that their child will become more rather than less upset by knowing what will happen. The child may become upset at first, but that upset should not be avoided; it is sometimes necessary to start the preparation process. In mild to moderate levels, this anxiety promotes coping with the new situation. If you avoid the task of preparing your child, being thrown into a new, scary, and possibly painful and distressing situation can negatively affect the child's health encounters for years—and not only those that occur in hospital.

If you choose not to say anything about going to hospital, why it is necessary, and what specifically will happen there, children invariably construct for themselves what the encounter may be like—it is a natural coping strategy. Having some realistic notion of the hospital encounter will counteract the spontaneous fantasies that most children experience when they draw on other children's graphic stories of hospital or on episodes in films or television clips. Some spontaneous fantasies can be far more anxiety-provoking than the reality of the hospital.

FITTING PREPARATION TO THE CHILD'S TEMPERAMENT AND NEEDS

Good preparation for dealing with pain begins with knowing your child's temperament, gathering some idea of her coping tendencies, and being open to her changing needs. Although a great deal is still not known about the interrelationship between children's temperaments and their coping abilities, mothers and researchers in child development have long known that even from the moment of birth there are differences in how newborn babies react, respond, and settle. Temperament is considered an innate, fairly stable characteristic of the child's personality. As the child grows and develops, temperament predisposes the child to a particular style of responding, a style that, research suggests, tends to remain consistent over the years; for example, the adaptable child tends to remains adaptable, and the high-strung child tends to react intensely, whatever his age.

Knowing your child's temperament can enable you to fit the preparation more appropriately to the child. For example, seven-year-old Susie, who needed surgery to remove the pencil tip from her cheek, was a bright, sensitive child, but she was not highly adaptable (adaptability is a key temperamental aspect of a child's capacity to "get ready" for a medical or surgical procedure). She needed time to let the news sink in that she had to have surgery to remove the pencil tip from her cheek. Fortunately, the hospital staff could be adaptable, and the procedure was performed one week later.

Some children say that knowing procedural details gives them a sense of control, whereas others say that it makes them anxious. Even within the same family, children (and adults) have different needs when attempting to cope. For example, a father may need detailed information to organize himself to deal with a stressful situation, whereas his child may make it clear that he does not like hearing the details and would rather his parents did not refer to the upcoming event at all. Most children, however, do want some idea of what to expect. If possible, ask the child how much he or she wants to know.

FITTING PREPARATION TO A CHILD'S AGE

Children's developmental differences also need to be taken into account when preparing them for hospital. Younger children are best prepared to cope with hospital procedures by creatively and spontaneously playing with a child's version of a doctor's kit in order to become accustomed to medical equipment, such as stethoscope, tourniquet, injections, bandages, and Band-aids. To develop coping skills, younger children tend to play out the actions of what may happen. In contrast, children older than eight and teenagers will tend to ask questions, require drawings and more detailed explanations, and engage in thoughts, fantasies, and images to prepare for and cope with hospital procedures. Teens often also require more complex explanations, and, unlike eight- to ten-year-old children, they tend to process and manage the situation on their own. The specific preparations that children of different ages require are covered in greater detail later in this chapter.

About Coping
COPING AT DIFFERENT TIMES

Research on children's coping ability is a new and growing field; the theoretical understanding of the different styles of coping has been drawn from adult studies. A key concept from this research is that coping is highly specific to each situation. For example, the same child may cope with a school test in one way and with a test of her hearing within a hospital environment in another. The meaning of the test and her appraisal of the situation—that is, how well she judges herself to be up to the test situation—are critical factors in determining how she will cope. A child's tendency to recognize a particular situation as stressful will vary greatly, depending on the child's age and stage of development, since each carries its own tasks, sensitivities, and challenges.

What is stressful for an infant in hospital, such as separation from parents, may not be as stressful for an 11-year-old or a 16-year-old. Similarly, adjusting to a splint on an arm or hand may not be as traumatizing for a 2-year-old as for a self-conscious 14-year-old, who wants to have more control over his world.

HOW CONTROL AND COPING AFFECT EACH OTHER

We know from research on adults that the greater the threat posed by a situation, the less control a person feels, and in turn, the less likely the person is to draw on coping strategies and the more likely he is to handle the stressful situation poorly and to become further distressed. Being distressed makes everyone feel a loss of control, and this negative cycle continues, further eroding confidence and motivation as the mishandled experiences add up.

Alternatively, if a person feels some control, the threat is diminished. An example of control is the ability to say to a physician during a procedure, "Please stop; I need to catch my breath!" This person is more likely to be able to make good use of coping strategies and consequently feel less distress and feel better about the experience and people involved. Explore with the physician or other health professional what control the child does have, how it could be spoken about, when it could be used, and what her choices are in this situation (for specific options see the section on control in chapter 6).

YOUR CHILD'S COPING

How a child has responded in the past to information that aroused anxiety and uncertainty can suggest how your child may cope in hospital. Ask yourself how your child approached other scary experiences, such as going to the dentist or doctor for the first time: Was she curious and questioning? Did she avoid any talk about the event? When you told her what was about to happen:

- Did she become concerned and check every possibility, becoming increasingly anxious, imagining worse scenarios as time went by?
- Did she soak up the information and immediately ask for more information, in a deliberate, searching manner, as if having the answers helped?
- Did she seem to downplay the information? If you stopped talking about the event and allowed her to come to you with questions, was she ready for a little chunk of information at a time? Did she deal with it well but in a low-key manner?
- Was telling her like meeting a blank wall, as if she didn't want it to happen and thought she could stop it from happening by not hearing anything about it? If you raised the matter again, did she reluctantly ask for basic information only, clearly not wanting the full details?

Answering these questions can help you understand how your child copes with anxiety and uncertainty. Keep in mind that one way is no better than another. This knowledge will help you understand how much information the child can comfortably handle at one time.

If you answer yes to question 1, your child can be considered a catastrophizer; yes to question 2 indicates a sensitizer; yes to question 3 indicates a minimizer; and yes to question 4 indicates a denier (see Figure 12.1).

|_____|_____|_____|_____|
Catastrophizer   Sensitizer   Minimizer   Denier

Figure 12.1 Coping Styles

Catastrophizers and Sensitizers

A sensitizer's way of managing uncertainty and anxiety is to collect detailed information. Sensitizers are most comfortable following this dictum: "The more I know about it, the better I can manage."

Carried to an extreme, this pattern can become what is called catastrophizing: information is collected, but it doesn't settle the child's anxiety. As his anxiety climbs, the child asks more and more questions, and the replies are not experienced as reassurance. The signs that the child's anxiety is running amuck are that the child tends to blow the details out of proportion and is overwhelmed and terrified by the information. Catastrophizers in a situation tend to think: "This is a total disaster and will never work out."

They tend to focus on the negative effects of pain: "I hate shots. That will hurt so much—it'll kill me!" They imagine unlikely negative consequences—"I'll never leave this hospital!"—and think about escaping and avoiding the procedure—"I wish my Dad would get me out of here now."

Such patterns of catastrophizing are also very common in children who have previously had bad pain experiences in doctors' clinics and hospitals and have not yet had any opportunity to discuss and resolve their experiences so that they can cope better on subsequent occasions. Often play therapy for younger children and pschyotherapy for older children, geared toward decreasing anxiety and developing adequate coping skills, is helpful.

Minimizers and Deniers

In contrast, children who are minimizers tend to play down the information as a way of coping with their anxiety and uncertainty. They put the potentially threatening information aside and privately digest it in small chunks and in their own time. When ready, these children will come back and collect specific information to address only specific concerns. Generally, these are children who function best not knowing it all, and need only the highlights.

Carried to an extreme, this style results in children who deny—that is, they totally push out of their minds the unpleasant experience with which they're going to have to deal. One way a denier copes with heightened anxiety is to say: "Don't remind me of it; I don't want to think or talk about it!"

This way of coping is not as common in children as it is in adults. Denying, like all the coping styles, is a way of protecting oneself; but that style isn't necessarily helpful when the person is confronted with the situation. You can help deniers by giving the key pieces of information orally and then leaving written information or returning to the topic in spaced chunks of time. Once again, psychotherapy can be a helpful process, preventing deniers from feeling too overwhelmed by the threatening information.

HOW COPING CAN CHANGE

It is worth repeating that there is no one way of coping that is right or wrong. The style or tendency of coping, like the personality of your child, is her individual way of dealing with the world and may be modified over time by learning, life experiences, parents' examples, and other influences. Children at the extreme ends of the continuum on the figure seem, however, to have higher anxiety and consequently to have a harder time coping with new or challenging experiences.

It is not uncommon for children to shift along the continuum and for a child who is normally a minimizer or a sensitizer to experience some denying or catastrophizing thoughts when he experiences a very frightening situation. In other words, a child's coping tendency is not static; as situations change, so does the child's way of coping.

If your child is having difficulties in coping and, for example, has persistent and overwhelming catastrophizing thoughts and fantasies, therapy with a child psychotherapist, child life worker, or nurse skilled in this area can help the child and family learn more adaptive ways of coping with hospital fears and experiences. Without therapeutic intervention, it is unlikely that your child's own naturally occurring style will change dramatically.

SPONTANEOUS COPING STRATEGIES

Some children, without any instruction, develop their own effective ways of coping. These can be thoughts that they say to themselves (self-talk, such as "I can do it"), memories or images that they draw upon, the reinterpretation of pain in a positive way ("This pain means that the tissues are knitting together so that I'll be able to go home more quickly"), or experiences they spontaneously re-create, like the earlier example of Kevin, who imagined himself as a wet noodle so that he would be comfortably relaxed before his spinal tap. Many children are ready to help themselves manage and get through pain and discomfort.

Preparing Children of Different Ages for Hospital
INFANTS

For infants, security is inextricably connected to Mom and Dad, and no formal infant preparation is needed before coming to hospital. What is crucial is preparation for parents. You will need to ask the following questions *before* going to hospital:

- What exactly is planned?
- What will occur in each procedure?
- How long does the procedure usually take?
- Who will be present, doing what?
- Can a parent be present?
- If a parent can be present, what would be helpful for you to do?

Ask for practical tips about what you can do to help the hospital visit go smoothly.

Gaining information in advance about the practical and procedural aspects of the hospital will help you to manage your own powerful feelings about taking your baby to hospital. Rather than gritting your teeth, inwardly seething, or resisting the procedure, take the time to become emotionally prepared for what is going to happen or what is already happening. Talk to your family physician, the nurse, or the social worker, psychologist, or child life worker on the ward to get you past any distress or anger you may feel that "all this is happening to my baby." Hospital staff are familiar with and sympathetic toward the natural and powerful feelings of distress, rage, and confusion that arise when a baby is ill.

- Stay as calm as possible as you focus on your baby. Infants are emotionally attuned to their parents' emotions: a parent's anxiety before going to hospital is quickly transmitted to the baby, who in turn becomes unsettled.
- Write down your baby's preferences for soothing and comfort, how she likes to be held, patted, or rocked, and remember to tell your hospital worker.

- Wherever possible, request to stay with your baby. Your voice, touch, and presence are immediate sources of reassurance and ease. Infants up to the age of five or six months will accept unknown caretakers. Older babies, however, will often show "stranger anxiety" and will be less tolerant of being handled by an unknown caretaker or being separated from parents.
- Familiar lullabies or music tapes and mobiles from home will provide familiar comfort. Such physical and emotional support helps your baby regain her equilibrium.

TODDLERS
Preparation
Toddlers (12 months to 24–30 months) understand the world in the here and now through direct body experiences and through a perspective centering on self. Children under two and a half years cannot make sense of a lot of preparation and can only grasp the events that they have experienced. Your little one may be bewildered and confused when asked to think about a future that he has not experienced. Unless the toddler has had previous hospital experiences, preparation before going to hospital will have limited effect.

- The key to making hospital manageable for toddlers is ensuring that the experience is as pain-free and as comfortable as possible, with the continuing contact and presence of attentive, loving parents.
- Preparation could be action-based and playful, using objects that are not the child's favorite playtoys to play out the scene.
- Introducing the subject at home will establish some concept of the procedure for your toddler. Note, however, that playing with a doctor's kit at home and being in the bewildering world of a hospital with painful needles are a world apart; thus, having some concrete familiarity with what will happen, with which part of his body, and why it will make life better is a helpful start for a toddler.
- What simple preparation you provide should take place shortly before going to hospital, no earlier than the day before, and again on the day of the hospital visit.
- Toddlers live marvelously in the here and now, so, for instance, if your toddler is going for elective surgery to repair a cleft palate, you could simply say: "Bunny is having her lip fixed here [point]. We're also going to hospital to have your lip fixed. Mommy and Christopher together. Here, Bunny, let's put a bandage on it. Your lip is getting

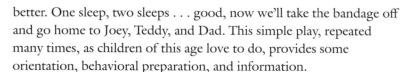

better. One sleep, two sleeps . . . good, now we'll take the bandage off and go home to Joey, Teddy, and Dad. This simple play, repeated many times, as children of this age love to do, provides some orientation, behavioral preparation, and information.

- Taking Bunny along, using the same language and action when you're in the hospital, and continuing and adapting the play can be enormously reinforcing and reassuring for your toddler. You're helping to make sense of the experience as it unfolds.
- Repeating the experience symbolically through play establishes a comfortable support and alliance between parents and child. Your child is likely to become less anxious, be more cooperative, and have a better experience.
- Take along a favorite comfort toy, security blanket, and other distracters, such as bubbles for blowing and favorite storybooks. These playthings can be combined with comforting reminders or phrases that you use at home to help offset the surprise and distress of an examination, procedure, or surgery—for example, "Let's rub to get the owie to go. Now it's all over and the Band-aid is on."
- Some clinics and hospitals have videotapes to prepare children of different ages for particular procedures or surgery. Watch these first and determine if your toddler would be helped by viewing them. Discuss with the hospital staff, particularly the child life worker, if they have other materials, such as puppets specifically designed for preparing toddlers for the medical or surgical intervention.
- The best preparation for first-time exposure of toddlers and infants going for surgery or procedures is for you to be well prepared and outwardly calm and collected about what your little one will go through. Indeed, parents' presence and comfort are the best source of comfort and preparation for all ages.

Tips for painful procedures
- Emphasize the end of the procedure with a phrase such as "It is all finished!" or "It's over!" Incorporate this into the preparation play as the sign that the procedure or examination has come to an end, so that it becomes a ritual. I recall a two-and-a-half-year-old with leukemia who, after playing with his doctor's kit and jabbing any stuffed animal in reach multiple times with the syringe, would chime out, "It's all over. No more today!" He knew and was comforted by such limits—however much the needles bothered him, they would end.

- Band-aids carry magic properties for many children. If Band-aids are a part of the procedure, announce with pomp and drama, "Now's the time for the Band-aid!" Toddlers undergoing repeated procedures will often insist on holding the Band-aid as security that the procedure will end.
- If possible, allow your toddler to move, walk, run around, or get involved with physical play as soon after the procedure as possible. His natural motor activity works off distress and restores some normality.

PRESCHOOLERS
Preparation

For preschool-aged children (three to five years), doing some things by themselves is a thrill; they derive a sense of accomplishment and self-esteem from taking initiatives.

- Preparation could be structured around a series of tasks for the child, as long as she is able to understand and follow clear direction, and likes to be able to help. The mastery of the first task can carry the child on a high to the next and on through the whole experience. Noticing and complimenting your child on whatever she has accomplished strengthens coping skills. For example: "You worked really hard at keeping still as the tourniquet went on. I saw that. It helped. Good work!"

With preschool and older children, a few more issues come into play:

- What the timing of information should be
- What type of procedural information would be interesting, helpful, and non-threatening to your child (if you're not sure, check with the hospital staff)
- What coping method would help your child during the new uncertain situations on the ward or during medical procedures

Preschoolers do best when they are prepared three to five days before going to the hospital. Even for a serious medical intervention, such as surgery, five days ahead is time enough for the younger child. More than five days is a very long stretch if hospital talk is to be the major topic of conversations. If the preparation begins too soon, the process could backfire, and the child could become anxious and preoccupied with concerns about going to the hospital. Three to five days before a procedure or surgery is generally enough time to mobilize coping skills and to rehearse, plan, and play to make the experience manageable.

Tips for painful procedures with preschoolers

With your child's temperament and coping tendencies in mind, plan your preparation. Here are some options for preschoolers:

- Play out the procedure using three-dimensional objects or non-favorite toys. (Children often imbue their favorite stuffed toys with feelings, and the possibility of its being hurt in any way will arouse the child's anxiety and bring out protective reactions.) Physically handling the objects is an essential part of the learning. Information conveyed in the play includes what the child will see, hear, or feel as body sensations and what he may be expected to do, such as lie curled up "like a pussy cat" to allow access to the spinal column for a tap.
- Look at pictures and diagrams with a simple explanation about what will happen, and you can also draw rough sketches. Your child can then draw a picture herself for a sibling or friend to explain what is going to happen and how she will feel when it's all better.
- Rehearse coping methods, such as counting or deep breathing to relax, storytelling, or using imagery or music to transform the situation (for elaboration, see chapter 6).
- Visit the hospital ahead of time, see the ward, and say hello to the staff.
- If relevant, provide comforting reminders of previous hospital successes to support your child's confidence.
- Minimize the procedural details (such as needles), and make note of the landmarks: "Remember when you see the blood flowing there'll be no more owie!"
- Maximize the support: provide a favorite tape or toy, or ask a grandparent to accompany you and your child.
- For needle procedures, give the child a Band-aid to hold as a way of ensuring that the procedure will come to an end. The Band-aid also means that the hurt will be fixed. Years ago I asked a four-year-old bright spark, "How come Band-aids are so wonderful?" He bluntly told me, "Band-aids make the hurt better and it makes it heal quick." I had to pursue this further: "That's wonderful . . . how does it do that?" "It fixes it, don't you know!" So I learned!

SCHOOL-AGED CHILDREN

Preparation

Here are some ways to prepare school-aged children (7 to 12 years) for hospital:

- Discussing, reading, and jointly preparing coping plans can begin within a week before the hospital procedures and investigations. With older children you are the best judge to determine how much time your child needs to get his mind in gear, to quiz you or his doctor, or speak to someone else who has had the same experience to help make sense of the hospital, procedure, or surgery.

- At this age, children can anchor their experiences in more logical, concrete ways than younger children, and fantasy plays a less significant part. Therefore, explanations about how the body works, why the procedure or surgery is needed, and briefly what will occur can be helpful in providing a conceptual framework for your child to organize her thoughts and apprehensions.

- Do, however, pay attention to your child's fantasy explanations for the hospital encounter. If the fantasy reflects any distortion or misconceptions of the experience, you may wish to clarify them, to help your child manage his fears. The child might, for example, be confusing pain with punishment: "I have to have those needles because I did something wrong." It is worth listening to your youngster's spontaneous play and talk so that you can prevent any further misunderstandings.

- Since school-aged children have a more developed understanding of time, they are better able to relate the hospital experience to the past, present, and future, and they have a sense of a future beyond the hospital event.

- Children of this age have a more accurate sense of their bodies than do younger children, and some can feel a correspondingly greater sense of personal threat or fear of body mutilation. If your child has these fears, look at pictures and body diagrams with clear explanations about the procedure and use other hospital materials, pamphlets and information, such as X-rays. You could draw a body outline (using Figure 5.6) and depict what you understand will happen, how his body could feel, and how it will recover. Or you can ask the surgeon, physician, or nurse to run through the process again for your child. Note that these explanations will not always dispel anxiety but will enable your child to manage any anxiety better by having a more accurate notion of what is to occur.

- Keeping up with her peers and developing a sense of competence with her peer group is important to the school-aged child. If appropriate for your child, talking or rooming with a similarly aged child undergoing a similar experience can be very helpful in providing camaraderie and can assuage the child's feelings about being different: "So I'm not the only one in the world with a kidney problem!"

- Plan to bring in favorite board games, toys, or video games.
- As with all age groups, it is best for you to prepare yourself for your youngster's hospital encounter apart from your child so that you are free to question and explore all the possibilities without having to concern yourself with the impact of this discussion on your child. The opportunity to examine every aspect to your satisfaction will free you to support your child more fully when he is in hospital.

Coping style and a working alliance

With school-aged children and teens a cooperative working alliance between child, parents, and staff is often crucial to successfully perform a painful procedure. Drawing on the coping style of your child can be helpful in establishing a good working alliance. Also, by early school years, a child's coping style has become more evident and established.

1. If your child's coping tendencies are mostly those of a *catastrophizer*, present the procedure in a calming way, explaining why she needs to have this done. I've nicknamed catastrophizers "dramatists" since they have a great sense of the dramatic and can heighten their tension very quickly. Since catastrophizers' anxiety can quickly spiral out of control, settling this anxiety becomes the first task:

- Acknowledge up front that you know your child gets worried easily about going to hospital. Remind her that this is her way of coping.
- Ask her in a low-key and calm manner to consider how many catastrophes have actually happened, or encourage her to think of the very worst thing that could happen, then explore why that could never indeed happen in this case. (Although remember, fear is not necessarily logical, and you're not going to finally win the child over through logic. Nevertheless, raising some of these arguments against her fears will bring some hope into the child's mind and possibly help.)
- Add that you are not worried (and sound convinced) because it is, for example, a straightforward procedure or a non-invasive examination, or because she won't have any more needles, or it only takes 20 minutes, or 6 hours, and then she'll come home to sleep.
- Conclude by reassuring her that you or whomever she chooses will be part of a team to support the process, and you would like to work on some coping strategies that will help her stay cool and cope well.

2. If you have deduced that your child approaches tough new situations as a *sensitizer,* come prepared with books, charts, or videos, and even the phone number of another child who has successfully undergone the proposed procedure and will speak to your child about surviving it. Be prepared to talk or sketch the procedure out several times, and reiterate that now that he knows these details, he'll manage much better. Then talk about some of the behavioral and imagery strategies that you can use together.

3. If your child is more of a *minimizer,* have on hand one or two items of information that you can casually leave lying around the table and that she can browse through if she wishes. Encourage her to come back to talk about it again a little later. Break the information into manageable pieces when you talk; be careful of overwhelming your child, and if your child becomes uncomfortable, stop and reassure her that it'll be okay and there's time enough for her to digest what will occur.

4. If, however, you conclude that your child is the rare *denier,* tell him what he needs to know very matter-of-factly, if he'll stick around to hear it! If not, tell a friend on the phone when he is in the room, or discuss it with your spouse or other children at the table to inform them of what will happen, and how it will be manageable, so that he can take it in without feeling pinned down.

Tips for painful procedures

- Having and exercising choices is helpful for all children, particularly school-aged children. Providing what choice you can in situations where choices are usually limited can go a long way toward helping your child hold onto some sense of self-control and competency. Your child may choose which hand to be used for drawing blood, for example.
- Rehearse and draw on coping methods, such as storytelling or counting backwards from 100 in twos, or in a foreign language the child is learning, and practice and use breathing to release tensions during the procedure.
- Provide active coaching and comforting reminders of previous hospital successes of friends or family members to support your child's confidence.
- Children of this age group like to feel that they can manage to do some things on their own and derive a sense of accomplishment and increased self-esteem from these initiatives. Remember to compliment your child on whatever she has accomplished: "You held your hand so still. I saw that. It helped them get the blood sample quickly. Good work!"

- Choose your child's favorite comforting music for an audio-tape or Walkman, which can be played, if the child chooses, before, during, and/or after the procedure.
- In your concern that all go well for your child, be careful not to depict the hospital encounter as a "wonderful time" or promise that "everything will go well." Giving those guarantees can backfire, and everyone can feel let down. Be honest about some of the uncertainties and emphasize your trust in your child's healthy body and good healing and coping abilities: "You've got a strong, good body—you'll recover well!"
- Understand that even though your child may have become very independent, the strangeness of the hospital and procedures and his apprehensions can make the best-adjusted child clingy and needy. This regression is normal, and your presence, comfort, and reassurance are often the best remedy. As soon as your child is feeling well again, this dependent, anxious behavior often disappears.
- If your child is going to stay in hospital, remind her that she will be coming home. Even for ten-year-olds, time is experienced in the here and now. One way to mark the passage of time is according to how many sleeps it will be before discharge. Remember, however, that hospitals are environments in which things change very quickly: the date of discharge may be delayed or rapidly brought forward, depending on many factors, including the progress and improvement of your child. So in your prediction, err on the side of a longer stay.

ADOLESCENTS

Preparation

Substantial changes in thought processes, physique, and emotions mark the adolescent years (ages 13 to 18) as exciting and turbulent; they are also the beginning of a long transition into adulthood. Every health encounter can be a threat to the teenager's sense of self, safety, self-control, and emerging independence. During this time the teenager's ability to think through situations takes a quantum leap, as abstract thinking and reasoning skills develop.

- Discussing and reading about the procedure and jointly preparing coping plans can begin when you best judge so that your teenager has the time to quiz you, or his doctor, or to speak to someone else who has experienced what he will have to go through. Often you will notice your child or teenager mulling it over on his own. This is part of coming to terms with the forthcoming hospital encounter and its implications not only for his physical well-being but also for his social and emotional life. If your teenager is open to talking things over with you during a mulling time, it may provide another productive exchange; if not, acknowledge your willingness to talk when your teen wishes.

- Adolescents can never be told too many times that "we want you home" and that "you are coming home." Barbara, who had been hospitalized with polio in her early teens, said that from her experience what she needed was "to be listened to, taken seriously, reassured regularly, comforted, believed, and to be told repeatedly that I was not going to be abandoned. Lastly, I needed to be taught how to speak up!"

Tips for painful procedures

- At all costs do everything to preserve your teenager's dignity. One of the most prominent fears that teenagers have is "losing it" and either crying or reverting to "childish" behaviors. You can prevent this regression and sense of being overwhelmed by closely monitoring what's happening, what your teen needs by way of explanation, or offering emotional or physical support and active coaching. If your teen cries, reassure her that it is not a sign of failure and that this has indeed been a tough situation.
- Teenagers can underplay a situation by "being cool"; don't, however, underestimate their terror, which often can be seen in their eyes, mouth, and voice quality, and in the draining of color from their face.
- Do everything to promote the notion that your teenager is in charge of his body. For example, you might say: "You know your body best—is that feeling all right? Do you need more analgesic?" Self-reliance and self-management are key issues for teens.
- Before coming to hospital parents may need to negotiate what role their teenager wants them to take during the procedure: "Do you want me to remain in the room?" "Yeh, Mom, but don't do any talking, OK?" Whatever your teenager's decision, accept it. Your teenager needs to feel empowered in the disempowering hospital situation, and now is a good time to start.

RESOURCES FOR PREPARATION AND COPING

Many preparation videotapes, slide shows, booklets, puppet shows, and prop boxes are available through children's hospitals for a range of medical investigations, procedures, and surgeries. Some are made for parents, and others are for children or teenagers. Ask at your hospital, or contact the Association for the Care of Children's Health (see Recommended Resources for the address) for their resource list of books and audio- and videotapes. Many hospitals now have videotape facilities where you can watch educational tapes. Remember, however useful the preparatory information, it may be confusing to your child or teen. Therefore, first screen the material yourself and preselect sections, rather than inundate your child with more information than she may want to have. Because of your understanding and relationship with your child, you will know more clearly than others whether she will find the information useful. You may find it helpful to stop the tape periodically to discuss the information to ensure that it makes sense.

Resource materials are very useful for a number of reasons:

- They tell the story of what will happen in a child-centered and developmentally appropriate manner.
- They often include demonstrations of other children performing the necessary actions or undergoing the investigations or procedures. Such illustrations of how they coped provide good modeling for the viewing child or teen.
- They are realistic and provide an opportunity for the child to get used to what will happen while sitting in the comfort of a chair. This desensitization can reduce anxiety at the time that the procedure occurs.
- They explain the reason for the procedure in language that is easier to understand than the medical jargon the child will hear in the hospital.

Next Time: Returning To Hospital

For some children, being in hospital is not a one-time event. How the child regards the next visit and the proposed investigations, procedures, or surgery will largely depend on whether the previous experience in hospital was positive or negative.

WHEN THE PREVIOUS HOSPITAL EXPERIENCE HAS BEEN POSITIVE

If your child's hospital experiences have been positive and relatively pleasant, returning to hospital requires some discussion, planning, recapitulation of what worked and what did not work, and rehearsing of the best coping skills. Your child will benefit from reassurance that you have confidence in him that he can do it once again. Reassurance should be based on what indeed went well last time and what he did to help himself through it. It helps to know if a familiar hospital professional (such as your child's favorite nurse, blood technician, or physiotherapist) will be there. Determine:

- What exactly will be done on the visit.
- Who will do it (get name and specialty, if possible).
- How long it will take this time. Add another third to that estimate, because everything takes longer than expected in hospital.
- Plan a reward afterward so that your child can anticipate the treat.

WHEN THE PREVIOUS EXPERIENCE HAS BEEN NEGATIVE

Returning to hospital for children who previously experienced unexpected pain there, who were told that "it won't hurt" and then it did, or who were forcibly restrained evokes vivid memories of what happened last time. Younger children may not be able to verbalize their fears as older children might; nevertheless, parents will notice the pre-verbal child stiffening physically, clinging more than usual, or whimpering. A child only needs one negative experience to sensitize her and to feed fears about the next hospital encounter.

Pain is a rapid and powerful teacher—all one needs is one bad experience and it is uphill work for parents and hospital staff to regain the child's trust and for the child to become comfortable and relax. That trust can be regained, however, and with gentleness, persistence, therapeutic assistance, and desensitization, a child can recover and learn how to manage what he formerly found to be terrifying.

Survival Skills for Parents

As parents, part of being prepared is recognizing that events may not go as they are supposed to. There's no place like a hospital to test that one out! Hospitals are controlled chaotic environments where the unexpected often happens. Despite the best efforts of many people and services that have to coordinate and function interdependently, sometimes predicting when and how things will go is a gamble. The larger the hospital, the more challenging your task. The better you know the hospital section or unit, the nature of the procedures, and the necessary components of the treatment, the better off you'll be in predicting accurately. Therefore, before your child enters the hospital, figure out:

- What questions to ask, and to whom you should ask those questions.
- Who is a good back-up person to check what is or isn't happening.

Become as knowledgeable as possible about:

- What your child's nature, coping style, and needs are.
- What your child's medical condition and symptoms are.
- What examinations and procedures are to be done and why.
- Who provides the procedures and what is needed for them to occur.
- What each professional in the team can and should do.
- How and when medications should be administered.
- How and when re-assessment and follow-up should occur.

In short, you need to quickly become an expert and your child's best advocate. Keeping a notebook and jotting down the information as you piece it together is a wonderful survival skill.

After you have gleaned this information and entered the hospital, be as flexible as you can and encourage your child to go with the flow. This advice may seem like a contradiction, but it isn't. Hospitals must meet the multiple demands of the many other sick and distressed children and their families, all wanting to get better, and you must fit in.

GO WITH THE FLOW

Going with the flow does not, however, mean passively handing your child over to the hospital. It is, rather, a state of actively attending to what is happening, fitting in, and, if it is in your best interests, speaking up when there are pauses in the flow—which is the time hospital staff will be able to listen and do something differently for you. It is important to speak up if you think it necessary, because holding back causes resentment and frustration, both of which will take their toll on you, your child, and your relationships with your helpers. A good rule of thumb for gauging a situation in hospital is: go along with it when you can and when you sense that it is right. If, however, you determine that it isn't right and you can't go along, request a meeting for clarification or specific changes. The best way to think about how to speak up is to think of yourself as an advocate.

BE AN ADVOCATE

The role of advocate is speaking on behalf of your child, in your child's best interest, to ensure that your child is as pain-free and as well looked after as possible. This role may require you to give the verbal expression of your child's unexpressed distress, unhappiness, uncertainty, or despair. For example, if your child is tired and has had enough of visitors, you could say, "Jason is very tired right now. It has been a rough day for him. Would it be okay if you stayed very briefly or came back another day?" Although successful advocacy requires many judgment calls, including being sensitive to the hospital staff and the timing of your requests, some physicians have a great respect for patients and families who are active advocates for themselves and their children; they say that they find sessions with them enjoyable and stimulating, even if time-consuming.

It is important for parents to have trust in a hospital, but this trust must never be blind or unquestioning. Remember that you are the authority on your child. You know what she needs when she enters hospital, what will make her comfortable, what will shake her up or terrify her, what she needs to be able to cope. Don't allow shyness or personal differences to get in the way of speaking up for your child and yourself. Ask questions if procedures are unclear. Refuse to be intimidated by titles or attitudes of "you're getting in the way." You have the right to have your concerns and your questions addressed. You are entitled to have access to those responsible for your child's care, and you are a vital part of your child's treatment team.

BUILD WORKING RELATIONSHIPS WITH HEALTH CARE PROFESSIONALS

Build up reliable working relationships and alliances with the health care professionals attending to your child. Each professional has an individual response to a child, parents, and their requests, and many do become emotionally involved and invested in supporting your child's treatment and want to see a full recovery. The caring and the team work between parent and child, parent and staff, staff and family unit, parents and other parents, staff and volunteers, and staff and staff are an essential part of making the hospital stay manageable and effective.

REMEMBER THAT HOSPITAL TIME IS ELASTIC

Time often evaporates for health professionals in a hospital. Sometimes the time allocated to be spent with one patient gets gobbled up by another patient or an unscheduled event that demands immediate attention and involvement (here is the chaos factor at work again). To a clinician in a hospital, having enough time to do all that one needs and wants to do is a challenge, requiring exceptional time-management skills.

In contrast, for children and their families, time in hospital can drag. To help it shrink, bring along such items as books, music, Walkman and tapes, radio, puzzles, and games for your child to play with you and visitors—and if you're lucky, the occasional nurse on night duty. Note also whether there are parents' support groups, lectures, or a parents' resource library. These are some of the ways not just to survive your child's stay in hospital but to make it an opportunity to cope and even transcend difficult and demanding days.

In conclusion, preparing for and coping in hospital are continual and dynamic processes. However, without the support of a trusted adult, even the finest preparation may fall short. An unsupported child spends so much energy adjusting to the foreign situation that she has little energy left to obtain or absorb the necessary information.

CHAPTER 13

Pain from Medical Treatments

The "Ouchless Place"

Frequently children in hospital who need regular invasive painful treatments do not feel safe in their beds. A nurse can pop into the room at any time and say, "Time for another shot!" or "I have to take some blood." To prevent children from feeling on edge because of such practices, some children's hospitals have defined specific policies about where and how painful procedures must be done. At St. Francis Hospital in Hartford, Connecticut, the Department of Pediatrics has established a credo for the "ouchless place." When their child is admitted, parents are given a pamphlet (see figure 13.1) that describes the ward routine and promises that blood will only be collected at certain times and at a specific place—never at the child's bed. It also states that EMLA® will be applied beforehand, child life workers will help children through the discomfort, and a pain rating will be used for children after surgery to ensure that adequate pain relief is provided. This forward-thinking policy goes a long way to ensure that children can be as comfortable as possible during their painful medical treatments in hospital.

Many children's units have now formally made the child's bed a safe zone; if painful procedures need to be done, the child is taken to a designated treatment room on the ward. Although the child learns very quickly that the treatment room is the place where the painful things happen, and may as a result come to fear that room in particular, she also knows that her bed, the playroom, and other rooms on the ward are pain-free areas where she can feel safe.

Attempts have been made as well to defuse fear about the treatment room, making it as child-centered as possible. The room may have interesting posters on the wall or paintings or mobiles on the ceiling for the child who has to lie on his back. Books, bubbles, and some cuddly toys are available to absorb the child's attention before and during the treatments. Most important, the child is given the choice of having a parent by his side. Some centers are now actively encouraging children and their parents to acclimatize themselves to the room by reading stories, blowing bubbles, and stroking or massaging. Staff members talk soothingly to the child on the treatment table before the start of the procedure. (The staff should have already prepared the medical equipment before the child enters the room so that fears are not needlessly aroused, and the child should not be kept waiting.) In short, there is an increased awareness that a child-centered environment may help the child feel a little less frightened.

Parents in the Treatment Room

Each hospital department can have its own policy on whether or not parents are permitted into treatment or recovery areas. If children were asked, most would want their parents in treatment rooms for painful minor surgery. The child's interests are not the only ones to be considered in reaching this decision, however. Some medical practitioners are simply not comfortable performing painful procedures on children with their parents present, and consequently, the practitioners' comfort has tended to set the rule. Their arguments are that parents may become upset, faint, or get in the way of the procedure. Another reason, less admitted, is that these practitioners fear that their skill will be under scrutiny as they perform the procedure, making it more difficult for them to it carry out. This is particularly the case if the practitioner is in training, such as a medical resident, and is somewhat unsure of his or her technical ability.

Many hospital units have chosen to incorporate parents into the treatment of their children and to let parents choose whether they want to accompany their child for the treatment, particularly when treatments are frequent or recurrent, such as spinal taps, catheterization, removing a plaster cast, establishing a spinal epidural, drawing blood, starting an IV, or performing bone marrow aspirations. These units provide parents with the information necessary for them to make the decision whether they wish to be there or not.

In the oncology ward of B.C. Children's Hospital we came to a position that worked very well for all concerned. Parents were asked

How We Create an "Ouchless Place"

* We will try to draw blood only when absolutely necessary and at a single time during the day, reducing the number of "needle sticks."

* All blood work and procedures will be done in a special treatment room so that your child feels safe from pain in his or her own room.

* Whenever possible (when it is not an emergency), a local anesthetic cream will be applied one hour before blood work to minimize discomfort during the blood drawing.

* If a painful procedure is necessary, every effort will be made to keep your child as comfortable as possible. This may involve the use of behavioral approaches and/or the use of mild sedatives. Our main focus will be to keep your child free from pain and fear during the procedure.

* We encourage you to be present in the treatment room to comfort your child during a procedure. We will have toys and materials available for you to use.

* The hospital's child life worker is an expert in helping children cope with discomfort in the hospital and is available to you and your child if you have any concerns or would like some help in trying the techniques suggested here.

* If your child is secluded for surgery and requires pre-operative medication, we will make every effort to administer the medication in a pain-free way. If an intravenous line is required, we will try to make it pain-free, either with the use of local anesthetic cream or to place it when your child is already sedated.

* After the surgery is over, we will make every effort to keep your child comfortable through our pain management program. If he or she does have discomfort, just notify the doctor or nurse and we will modify the program until your child is comfortable. there is no reason why your child should be in pain after surgery.

* We use pain ratings in our program that are appropriate for your child's developmental level. You or you child may be asked to rate the pain so that adequate pain relief can be provided.

whether they wanted to accompany their child into the treatment room; if they said yes (a large majority), they were then told what the procedure entailed and what their role was as their child's ally and given a chair on which to sit. The chair was placed at the child's head, enabling the parent to focus on the child's face and to hold hands if desired—in short, to maintain close, comforting contact with the child. We encouraged parents not to focus on the technical part of the procedure; we would announce the various stages of the procedure so that they knew what was going on.

The parents' job, which they could do better than anyone, was to support, coach, and encourage the child to cope. We found that integrating the parent in this way into the child's treatment was invariably successful. Parents appreciated the involvement, and although being in the room was not always easy for them, they tended to be supportive of the medical and nursing team. (The parents' role in the cancer treatment of their child is depicted in the videotape *No Fears, No Tears*; see Recommended Resources.)

The staff also supported those parents who found the process of accompanying their child for a painful procedure too taxing. Some parents chose instead to come in halfway through the treatment, or after the worst part of the procedure was over, to comfort and to be with their child. The goal is to serve the best interests of the child and the parents, and the staff must remain flexible and open to necessary changes, particularly when the procedures are recurrent.

Policies in the recovery room, following anesthetic and surgery, are less flexible and more formal than in treatment rooms. The majority of children's hospitals (although there are some notable exceptions, such as the Children's Hospitals in Boston and at Yale) do not yet allow parents into the recovery room while the child is still unconscious and being monitored after surgery. As soon as the child is awake, however, if the child requests her parent or is very distressed, the recovery room nurse will fetch the parent to be with the child, who feels groggy and confused and needs a familiar, loving presence to provide security while reorienting to consciousness.

The Dreaded Needle

Needles are used to draw blood and fluids for investigations, to access skin, tissue, and veins to deliver medication and fluids, and often to administer analgesics to relieve pain. When children are asked what they associate with hospital, the large majority will say, "Needles . . . and the pain of needles." From a child's point of view, there are few worse ways to deliver medical care than via the sharp point of a needle. It becomes the stuff of nightmares for children requiring frequent needles for monitoring diabetes or for cancer treatment.

Few children can accept this rationale: "You will feel a sharp pain so that the pain medication can get into your body so that the pain can go." Adults do not tolerate short-term pain for long-term gain much better. Adults who as children required hospitalization and experienced a long line of needles will faint or flee from a needle as quickly as any youngster. The use of needles in children's care clearly highlights a clash of philosophies between a child-centered humanistic perspective of medical and nursing care and the efficiency-driven medical technology that considers the long-term impact of medical care on children irrelevant. Since each is necessary for effective health care, one of the challenges of 21st-century child medical care will be meeting the needs of both.

Whenever possible, medications for children should be given by mouth rather than by injection. The needle is the last resort, when no other route is available. In this circumstance, determine from the staff if there is another possible route, and if not, what kind of needle is to be given, because some needles are a lot less painful than others. Intramuscular injections tend to hurt more than IVs; and after an IV is established in a vein, medications can be inserted into the line with no further pain to the child. In a hospital situation when regular treatment is required, an IV is better to have than IM injections three or four times a day. Some clinicians go even further and are on record saying that because of the many harmful effects of using needles with children, such as anticipating pain, the sharp pain itself, and the resistance, non-cooperation, and terror that needles cause, needles should be banned for use with children.

If time is not as critical and you know that your child will not react well to a needle, ask if the same medication is available in oral form. Oral medication doses are usually higher than the doses for injection because the capsule or tablet passes through the digestive system before it is metabolized into the bloodstream. Benefits and risks must be carefully weighed; a needle will relieve pain faster than oral medication, but is painful. If circumstances permit, child, parents, and health care professionals should discuss the two options.

Fortunately, in the future, needles may be used less and less in child health care. Changes in the pharmaceutical industry will begin to reflect an awareness that needles are traumatic. Recently there has been a push to investigate alternative routes of delivering medications to children. For instance, if analgesic medication is placed in a medication lollipop for a child in the recovery room after surgery, the child sucks the lollipop until it takes effect. The medication is rapidly absorbed through the mucosa in the child's mouth, the child becomes relaxed and drowsy, and the lollipop slips out of his mouth.

More tolerable than needles, although still not a favorite for children, are intranasal administration (absorption through the sensitive tissues of the nose) and rectal administration (rapid absorption through the rectal mucosa). Children prefer having medication administered topically through the skin (transdermally), or under the tongue (sublingually). If a needle has to be used, the subcutaneous needle technique of delivering medicine is slightly easier on the child. The advantage is that it can be placed under the skin easily, you don't have to search for a vein, and the medication flow can be easily stopped and started.

Nevertheless, needles remain a medical mainstay. Needles are efficient, they are relatively safe and they allow medication dosages to be measured fairly accurately for each child's weight, age, and condition.

PREPARATION FOR A NEEDLE

If having a needle is the only option, it is crucial that you gather the necessary information to help your child cope. Below are some of the different forms of needles and injections that children in hospital can experience. Determine from the following list what kind of needle will be given to your child.

- *Intramuscular injection* into a child's upper arm, thigh, or buttocks is used to deliver immunizations, analgesia, and other medications.
- *Local anesthetic* delivered with a small needle is used to anesthetize a small portion of your child's body that may need suturing or for an invasive procedure, such as a spinal tap or bone marrow aspiration.
- *Subcutaneous injection* uses a fine (butterfly) needle immediately under the skin for the slow infiltration of analgesia or other medications or fluids.
- A *butterfly* or larger-gauge needle is used to access a vein in the arm to draw off blood.
- A *small butterfly* needle is used to access a vein in your child's hand or foot (or scalp for an infant) so that medication or fluids can be fed directly into the blood system.
- A *small finger stick* is used to draw peripheral blood from the tip of your child's finger (or heel for an infant); the blood is collected in a small collection tube or placed on a slide to be examined microscopically.

Preparing the skin

The most sensitive part of the skin is the surface, which is well supplied by nerve endings.

- If you have an hour or more before the injection, use the local anesthetic cream EMLA®. Hospital staff will sometimes be willing to put the cream on before a decision whether or not to give a needle is reached.

- If EMLA® has not been used, you can briefly desensitize the child's skin by rubbing it briskly with your fingertips, or by placing an ice cube to temporarily numb the area immediately before the needle is inserted. Ice, however, provides only about three seconds of anesthesia. An ice cube cannot be used for an IV insertion since cold constricts veins, making access more difficult.
- Some centers will also use ethyl chloride spray, which briefly anesthetizes the surface of the skin. Feel free to inquire about what your nurse or physician plans to use to minimize the child's pain.

Establishing a helpful plan

Provide your child with a helpful plan by saying: "How about if you do your blowing right now and we'll see how that helps so that you're not bothered by the injection," or "Let's do (any of the coping techniques, such as counting, tightly squeezing a hand and letting the discomfort drain, or using a favorite image to soften the pain) so that you won't feel the discomfort nearly as much. Come, let's do it now." Or "You're the boss of your body; where should we go right now to help your body become so relaxed that you hardly feel the needle? Should we go snorkel in Hawaii, or would you rather go skiing?"

By combining physical pain-relieving strategies with your child's coping strategies, the amount of perceived pain decreases and the child will not be as shocked by the invasive procedure. Following are some specific strategies to help reduce discomfort with each type of needle or injection.

TYPES OF INJECTIONS
Intramuscular (IM) injection

Since the pain from an IM shot is a sharp jab, unprepared children are startled as the needle goes in. Further discomfort or stinging is often experienced as the fluid is infiltrated into the muscle tissue. Depending on the medication, a very small amount of fluid may or may not sting; a larger amount (1 cc or more) invariably will. The discomfort *may* be reduced if the fluid is infiltrated slowly, allowing it time to be absorbed into the tissue.

If your child needs or already has an intravenous line (IV) established, an additional IM shot should not be necessary, unless the medication cannot be given any other way. The IV can be used to deliver most medications. Discuss this with your nurse or physician. Since this injection is a short one, it is all the more important for your child to use a pain-coping strategy, such as blowing bubbles, rhythmic breathing out, or taking an imaginary journey before the injection. You must also actively support your child during the brief, sharp pain and continue the support after the injection is over, since the pain can persist for a while.

Local anesthetic

A local anesthetic injected through the skin into the tissue is used to numb surrounding tissue before minor surgery, invasive procedures, or suturing. This experience can be painful, scary, and upsetting for children of all ages. Some physicians will recommend that EMLA® be placed on the site 90 minutes before the procedure to numb the skin before the local anesthetic is infused.

The best way of preventing the local anesthetic from stinging is to used a buffered form. The local anesthetic is best infiltrated *slowly* into the tissue layers, and *a minimum of 3 minutes* must elapse after the infiltration for the anesthetic to take effect and numb the affected tissue. It is important that the local anesthetic be given enough time to become effective or the child will feel the pain of the procedure that follows.

Subcutaneous infiltration

This form of injection is generally used with chronically ill children in exceptional situations, such as when the ill child's veins are difficult to access and the child needs analgesic medication or extra fluids. A fine-gauge IV butterfly needle is placed just underneath the top layer of the skin in the upper arm or leg if it is a short procedure, or under the collarbone if an infusion is continuous or intermittent so that the body can absorb the medication or fluids. This is a very useful method for providing pain relief at home, when the child cannot swallow medication.

Blood work

This is the term used for drawing blood from a larger vein in the child's hand or arm (usually the crook of the child's elbow, where access to the veins is easiest). The blood technician will customarily use a rubber tourniquet on the upper arm to increase the blood pressure, which dilates the vein, providing easy access. The technician may also ask your child to pump her hand to further increase the pressure in the vein. As soon as the vein is accessed and the blood is flowing, the tourniquet should immediately be released.

The tourniquet is tight and can trouble children. Explain to your child beforehand why it is being used and how it can "help the veins to stand up strong." Your child can briefly play with the tourniquet to feel its stretch. To help your child get through this procedure with minimal discomfort, determine first what she would like you to do to help it go better, such as squeeze your hand or blow out. As soon as the tourniquet is on, actively coach your child to focus and use a coping method. If, for example, she selects blowing out, you can remind your child that it helps her body to feel good and encourages the veins to stand up. Blowing bubbles can also be helpful as a visual distractor for this short procedure, helping the child get through the moment of anticipating pain and the sudden pain itself. It also interrupts crying and enables the child to retain some dignity. Pay close attention to your child; your presence and encouragement are a powerful help. Provide reassurance, praise your child for her effort, and compliment what she did well. This sets up a positive memory for the next time blood has to be drawn, since the procedure may need to be repeated.

IV

To provide continuous access to the blood system for fluids or medication or to intermittently draw blood, a small-gauge needle, sometimes referred to as a butterfly needle, is commonly used. On each side of this small needle is a plastic flap that can be pinched together with the forefingers so that the needle can be stabilized and positioned into the veins of the hand, foot, or scalp. This procedure requires skill, particularly to identify the "good" veins in toddlers' plump little hands. The process of holding still and having a vein accessed is often stressful and painful for children. The procedure requires that the needle be carefully placed within the vein and not punctured through the vein so that the fluid drains into the surrounding tissue. Unfortunately, an IV is not always established in one attempt, and a second or third try may be required or another vein may need to be accessed. This is very wearing on children who desperately want it to be in and over.

Once it is established, the child's hand and arm must be stabilized with the IV in site. Commonly the IV will be taped to the skin to hold it in position, and the child's arm or foot may then be taped onto a small board to minimize any movement that could dislodge the IV.

To make it more manageable for your child:

- Determine that the person doing the IV has experience with IVs; there may be other, more suitable situations for a new trainee to gather experience. Since the introduction of EMLA®, which needs to be applied 90 minutes before the procedure, IV access need no longer be painful and distressing. There are some children who have become so terrified of needles that using the cream does not make the experience any easier.
- The finer veins on the hand or foot are more easily accessed when warm. Use a heating pad, water bottle, warm cloth, or your warm hand to dilate these veins. Gently rubbing the veins can also achieve provide warmth.
- The peripheral veins commonly contract with anxiety and fear, so once again it is important to keep your child engaged in actively coping.
- Most children like to watch the procedure to see what is happening. If your child so chooses, allow him to watch, since this is a good way for him to integrate and make sense of the process. Some parents fear that permitting their child to watch will be damaging and the child will become more fearful. We have found it important to let a child choose. Those children who elect not to look often know what is about to happen and prefer to distract themselves. With a first IV, a child, however young, will often watch the entire process intently, taking in every detail.

Finger stick

A small amount of blood is collected from the tip of a finger by using a small needlelike tool called a lancet. The blood that starts to ooze out may be collected on a slide for microscopic examination. It may also be collected in a hollow fine tube (a pipette) or a small collection tube for a blood sample. The tips of fingers are filled with fine nerve fibers and are exquisitely sensitive, however, and children's fingertips are even more sensitive than those of adults. In addition, children often find having their fingertips squeezed acutely uncomfortable.

Once again, it helps to temporarily numb the fingertip with ice and blow, or to desensitize the child's fingertip by briefly rubbing it. Unfortunately, pain-reducing methods are not often used for finger stick procedures. Hospital staff tend to regard finger sticks as minimally painful, yet children often detest them as much as they do any other needle procedure. Informing the blood technician of your plan to reduce this momentary discomfort will go a long way toward easing a child's visit in hospital, since finger sticks may be frequent and for some are a daily procedure.

Children requiring daily blood collection, such as children with diabetes, can learn to do this procedure themselves using a little automatic device. As they depress it on the fingertip, a fine needle darts out and quickly pricks the skin, drawing blood. If managing "by myself" is a big issue for your child, ask if this device is available.

Other Common Invasive Procedures

The other common invasive procedures that are done to children in hospital include catheterization, spinal taps, and endoscopies.*

URINARY CATHETERIZATION

In the absence of any pathology, the procedure of inserting a catheter (small connecting tube from the bladder that drains urine) into the urethra is an uncomfortable procedure but not necessarily a painful one. Because the catheter is placed in the child's genitals, the child can easily feel embarrassed or ashamed. An explanation, sensitively given, and some discussion will help prepare the child. Curtains must be drawn and respect for the child's feelings shown as the child lies down and is supported to remain still. Once again, the support person can activate the child's coping by using a favorite story, looking at a pop-up book, or breathing together while the catheter is put in place and the child's bladder is drained.

SPINAL TAP

A spinal tap or lumbar puncture is a neurological diagnostic test to determine intracranial pressure around the brain and spinal cord and to obtain a sample of cerebrospinal fluid, which can be useful for a variety of diagnostic tests, including checking for infection and bleeding. It can also be used to administer medication or anesthesia, such as a regional block before surgery. A fine long and hollow needle is inserted between

---

*Non-invasive diagnostic procedures such as X-rays, CAT scans, and EEGs can be very anxiety producing, but they are not painful. Nevertheless the same principles apply for enabling children to manage: adequate preparation, explanation, opportunity for discussion and questions, and provision of a supportive person to help them through the scary and strange experience.

the vertebrae in the lower part of the spine into the spinal canal (the subarachnoid space). A few millilitres of spinal fluid are drawn off into a sterile vial for analysis.

Before the procedure, your child will be asked to curl up into a fetal position, "like a kitty-cat," and a nurse will probably support her position. It is important that your child feel supported and not restrained or oppressed. Sedatives such as oral lorazepam, midazolam, or IV midazolam, can be helpful in cutting down your child's anxiety and discomfort. Midazolam administered through an IV will often disrupt the child's memory of the event so that after the procedure the child has poor recollection of what exactly happened. This can be a benefit, since the child then does not build up anxiety. Sometimes it can backfire, making the child feel out of control and confused. Other forms of conscious sedation can also be used, including nitrous oxide (laughing gas). It is useful to know what is available and used for sedation in your hospital.

GASTROINTESTINAL ENDOSCOPY OR COLONOSCOPY OR UPPER ENDOSCOPY

This investigation provides the gastroenterologist with a direct view of most of the gastrointestinal tract. Your child will need to be very well sedated or given a brief general anesthetic. This procedure is uncomfortable and a source of great embarrassment for most children. Thus, it needs to be very well handled to avoid both discomfort and shame. Parents are generally not permitted to be present during the procedure, which is considered a minor surgery procedure. You should be able to remain with your child until he falls asleep, however. A flexible fiber optic colon scope is gently introduced through the anal canal for the endoscopy, and through the mouth for the upper scope. Some air is introduced into the colon, which can cause discomfort. Photographs and biopsies can be taken with this instrument to help reach a diagnosis.

All of the common medical procedures described in this chapter are painful and therefore anxiety-producing for children. Parents need to ask the hospital staff for information about the procedure, what precisely occurs, how best to prepare the child, and how best to help the child cope.

CONCLUSION

PAIN IS MUCH MORE THAN a medical problem—it is part of everyone's life. Pain isn't just a matter of nerve synapses and neurotransmitters, or which analgesic should be used at what dosage. After years of neglect, pain is now being acknowledged as a problem in living. As such, it affects all aspects of the life of the person in pain and of those connected to that person. When that person is a child, a great amount of the responsibility to help assess and manage the pain rests on the shoulders of parents.

Parents are central to a child's well-being, and they guide and develop a child's attitudes toward, and behavior with, people, places—and pain. It is deeply shocking that we have overlooked the role parents can and do play, that we have neglected attending to children's early pain experiences, and that we have historically not provided adequate assessment and treatment of children's pain. Now that we know better, it is encumbent upon us to ensure that these old ways and old habits die and that our children have the pain relief and support they require, given by those who are most skilled at it—qualified, caring health care professionals and the child's parents.

Given their rightful role as their child's best ally, parents can ensure that thought and preparation goes into routine bloodwork, immunizations, examinations in medical clinics, dental procedures, and treatments in hospital wards. Responsible health care professionals must take action to ensure that parents are integrated into the required preparation and management. Parents have a deep understanding and bond with their children, one which can provide the strength and guidance to make sense of and manage pain, so that incidental pain or planned medical procedures and treatments no longer become a wounding, traumatic or phobia-inducing experience. Parents are now an essential part of the treatment team any time that a child is in pain.

I am frequently asked whether I think that a child who uses psychological pain management techniques feels the same amount of pain as a child who isn't using them. My reply usually is: If the child feels okay or even good about how her or she is handling a difficult situation, then it becomes a better experience compared with panicking or being flooded by fears and feelings of inadequacy. The pain is there, but the perception and relationship to it changes as the child engages in the coping technique. As a result, the amount of pain is experienced differently. One's perception, attitude, and behavior governs the experience—and therefore governs one's physiological reaction.

In the years ahead, as our research continues and understanding of the complex pain processes grows, so must our appreciation of the immense influence that the brain has on the processing of pain perception. Ultimately, all pain is in the brain. Yet when we deal with attitudes to pain and the pain experience we're dealing with a paradox. The more you invite yourself to work constructively with the pain sensations, the less power it has. The less power it has, the less it unsettles you or wrecks your life.

Thus the next neglected area of pain management to be seriously addressed will be a child's thoughts, attitudes, beliefs, images, memories and the current meaning of the pain. These are key components to improving pain management at home, in clinics and in hospital.

We are clearly more than a bundle of nerve fibres and neurotransmitters. As soon as a child feels pain or begins to fear pain parents and health care professionals must address how the child is perceiving, thinking, and responding to it. Harnessing children's attention, imagination, and concentration skills through coping techniques like imagery, breathing, relaxation, and hypnosis will transform a feeling of being victim to one of accomplishment. Through the development of this cognitive control—or brain power—the child or teen in team work with staff and loved ones begins to gain mastery in living with the body he or she inhabits.

Psychological methods, however, are no substitute for analgesics when such medication is needed, just as analgesics or sedatives are no substitute for talking to a child, addressing the child's fears, and mobilizing the child's coping ability. Analgesics, sedatives and other pharmacological agents are best in combination with attention to the child's thoughts and behaviors. Together, medications and coping methods dove-tail, one enhancing the effectiveness of the other. Opioid medications, for example, bring greater relief for a child who is receptive and actively relaxing and letting go. The child's pain relief will be even further enhanced by focussing his or her mind on pleasant images and thoughts, noticing the easing of the pain, distancing from the pain, or shrinking it, rather than fighting against it or being tense and anxious.

Pain touches many aspects of a child's life. If pain's touch is brief and light, a child may not be left with lingering fears. But at some point in their lives a significant number of children (approximately 15 percent of school-aged children) will have recurring or chronic pain. Pain marks these children's lives, as well as the lives of their parents and siblings. It alters their nerve fibers, changes how they experience themselves, and affects how they are able to live at home, at school and with their friends. At a conference in Italy in 1994, a multidisciplinary group of pain professionals, together with the World Health Organization, drew up a set of guidelines for the management of children's cancer pain. These recommendations are applicable to children's pain associated with many other diseases, such as sickle cell disease, arthritis, kidney and heart disease, and AIDS. The group recommended that:

- The joint use of pharmacological agents with psychological coping methods must be part of treatment from the time of diagnosis throughout the treatment process.
- Pain must be assessed regularly throughout the course of treatment.
- Adequate analgesic doses must be administered "by the clock"—that is, at regular times, and not when the child is in pain and requests relief.
- Analgesics should be provided "by the mouth" and painful routes of administration avoided whenever possible.
- A child's pain severity determines the level of analgesics and a step-wise approach following the WHO analgesic ladder (from mild analgesic to stronger, then to opioid) for selecting pain-relief drugs should be followed.
- Sufficient analgesic doses should be provided to allow children to sleep throughout the night, and side effects should be anticipated and treated aggressively.
- Parents and families are a vital part of the treatment team and need to be involved throughout the treatment process.

It is harder to encourage a child to cope when he or she is feeling ill, fatigued, scared, or in pain. Hence, a focus of this book has been to use the minor pain experiences of everyday life as opportunities to train a child to become "pain-literate." Literacy means the child can interpret the pain signal intelligently, rather than being overwhelmed by the fear of pain, and can accept support and be willing to help in letting the pain go. If we wait until the child is sick in hospital, it is uphill work, similar to learning to swim by being thrown into the deep end of a swimming pool. There are better and smarter ways than sink or swim. Our children deserve the chance to become competent and unafraid of dealing with pain. We as a society now have the knowledge, skills, and resources to address the pain experienced by infants, children, and teenagers, and to provide the control and relief that is their right.

RECOMMENDED RESOURCES

Association for the Care of Children's Health (ACCH). An education and advocacy organization of parents, professionals in child health, and hospitals that promotes family-centered policies and practices, and holds conferences and workshops throughout North America. 7910 Woodmont Ave., Suite 300, Bethesda, MD 20814. Tel 301-654-6549; 800-229-1350, Fax 301-986-4553.

Accepting Your Power to Heal: The Practice of Therapeutic Touch by Doris Krieger. Bear and Co., Santa Fe, NM, 1993.

Atlantis: The Imagery Newsletter, edited by D.J. Gersten, M.D. A quarterly publication on using imagery for many problems. 4016 Third Ave., San Diego, CA 92103.

The Challenge of Pain: Exciting Discoveries in the New Science of Pain Control by Ronald Melzack and Patrick D. Wall. Basic Books, New York, 1983.

Children in Pain—A Study, Parts 1 & 2 on a 90-minute videocasette ($195). Directed by Leora Kuttner, the video covers issues and dilemmas in pediatric pain management within a children's hospital.

Children in Pain—An Overview, 30-minute videocassette ($89). Provides highlights from the original program. Suncoast Media, Inc., 12551 Indian Rocks #15, Largo, FL 34644. Tel 800-899-1008, Fax 813-587-7942.

Childhood Constipation and Soiling: A Practical Guide for Parents and Children by Minneapolis Children's Medical Center, Behavioural Pediatric Program, 2525 Chicago Ave., S. Minn., MN 55404 ($6.95 US).

Childhood Pain: Current Issues, Research and Management by Dorothea Ross and Sheila Ross. The first book to examine children's pain and its practice, and interview children about their experiences. Urban and Schwarzenberg, Baltimore and Munich, 1988.

The Culture of Pain by David Morris. A compelling and scholarly book on cultural attitudes and pain practices current and historic. Berkeley University of California Press, 1991.

Help Yourself by P.J. McGrath, S.J. Cunningham, M.A. Lascelles and P. Humphreys. A first-class self-help program for migraine and tension headaches with one booklet for professionals ($9.95 Can.) and another for children ($19.95). University of Ottawa Press, 603 Cumberland, Ottawa, ON K1N 6N5.

Home Remedies for Children by Prevention Magazine Health Books. A useful reference book covering ailments from animal bites to warts. Rodale Press, Emmaus, PA, 1994.

Healing Visualizations: Creating Health Through Imagery by Gerald Epstein, M.D. Provides well-tailored imagery exercises for medical problems. Bantam Books, New York, 1989.

Hypnosis and Hypnotherapy with Children by Karen Olness and Daniel Kohen. The pre-eminent book on the subject; easy to read with rich clinical vignettes. Guilford Press, 1996.

Imagery in Healing by Jeanne Achterberg. An intelligent examination of how mind and body function as a unit, and how imagery is the golden thread of change. New Science Library, Boston, 1985.

Managing Pain Before It You by Margaret A. Caudill, M.D., Ph.D. A workbook for adults dealing with chronic pain, and could be useful for adolescents. Guilford Press, New York, 1995.

No Fears, No Tears: Children with Cancer Coping with Pain. A videotape (29 minutes) and manual made for parents and children with cancer ($60) by Leora Kuttner, Ph.D. Canadian Cancer Society, Education Dept., 565 W. 10th Ave., Vancouver, BC V5Z 4J4. Tel 604-872-4400.

Parents of Children with Chronic Illness or Disability by Hilton Davis. A helpful and well-written book. British Psychological Society, 1993.

Pain by Howard Fields. An erudite book on the physiology of pain. McGraw-Hill, 1989.

Pain in Children. Nature Assessment and Treatment by P.J. McGrath. An in-depth and sophisticated read for professionals and parents. Guilford Press, New York, 1990.

Pain in Infants, Children and Adolescents, edited by Neil Schechter, Chuck Berde and Myron Yaster. The most comprehensive and thorough book for professionals on all aspects of pain assessment and current treatment methods. Williams and Wilkins, 1993.

Pain, Pain, Go Away: Helping Children with Pain by P.J. McGrath, G.A. Finley and J. Ritchie. A booklet (15 pages) on understanding and managing children's pain. ACCH, 7910 Woodmont Ave., Suite 300, Bethesda, MD 20814. Tel 301-654-6549; 800-229-1350.

Pain in Children and Adolescents by P.J. McGrath and A. Unruh. A comprehensive textbook on the history, nature, and different forms of children's pain. Elsevier, Amsterdam, 1987.

Pediatric Diagnostic Procedures by Susan Droske and Sally Francis. Provides information on a wide range of medical tests in hospitals and detailed guidance for preparing children. Wiley Medical, New York, 1981.

The Puzzle of Pain by Ron Melzack. The classic book, first published in 1964, that opened new ways of understanding and treating pain.

Science of Breath: A Practical Guide by Swami Rama, R. Ballentine, M.D. and A. Hymes, M.D. An easy to read book for the lay-person on the function of the nose and chest in breathing and methods of breathing. Himalayan International Institute of Yoga Science & Philosophy, RR1, Box 400, Honsdale, PA 18431.

A Sigh of Relief: The First-Aid Handbook for Childhood Emergencies by Martin Green. A popular book with illustrations of what to do in common childhood emergencies. Bantam Books, 1984.

Spinning Inwards by M. Murdock. An excellent resource book on using imagery with children. Shambhala Publications Inc., Boston, 1987.

Standard First Aid and Personal Safety. American Red Cross manual available at offices throughout the United States.

A Standard Medical Release for your child is available from Communications Dept., McNeil Consumer Products Co., Camp Hill Road, Fort Washington, PA 10934.

Strategies: A Practical Guide for Dealing with Professionals and Human Service Systems by Craig V. Shields. An excellent guide to survival skills within a hospital. Human Services Press, Richmond Hill, ON, 1987.

St. John's Ambulance Manual. Available at St. John's Ambulance Offices throughout Canada.

Taking Charge: The Challenges of Long Term Illness by Irene Pollen, MSW and Susan K. Galant. Gives a helpful focus on chronic pain for a family. Times Books, 1994.

The Tragedy of Needless Pain by R. Melzack. An article on the undertreatment of pain. Scientific American, 262, #2, 1990, pp. 27–33.

Unlocking the Secrets of Pain: The Science, The Psychology, The Treatment—A New Era by Allan Basbaum. A compelling chapter on the history and latest information on pain. Encyclopeidia Brittanica, 1987, pp. 84–120.

Where the Mind Meets the Body by H. Dienstfrey. A fascinating read on how mind and body interact in illnesses. Harper-Collins, New York, 1991.

Window to Our Children by Violet Oaklander. Explores understanding children through art, fantasy, and play. Real People Press, 1978.

Your Child's Health by Barton Schmitt, M.D. A well organized parent's guide to symptoms, emergencies, common illnesses, behavior and school problems.

~~ ACKNOWLEDGMENTS

IN THANKING THE PEOPLE who have helped make this book come to life, I am reminded of the series of jokes about how many people it takes for a particular profession to change a light bulb. My discovery was how many people it takes to write a book: one to sit in solitary and write— and at least 45 others to discuss, question, inspire, read wisely, support, answer questions, re-read and share in the experience of the emerging form. I am indebted to all and wish to thank:

My marvellous husband Tom, who picked up the considerable household slack when this book came to live and grow in our home. He encouraged, advised, untangled computer glitches and did wonders. My two children Tamar and Daniel, who with delightful humour and candor added many insights into how children think, deal with and interpret pain. They shared the computer with me— not once accidentally wiping off anything. Dr. Dorrie Ross who reminded me for a number of years that there was a book that needed to be written for parents on children's pain and urged and encouraged me to write it. To Jack and Dr. Selma Wassermann who pointed me in the right direction.

My five colleagues who contributed to the book: Dr. Barbara Shapiro, a Pediatrician who spent many years as co-director at Children's Hospital of Philadelphia Pain Clinic, gave generously of her time, attention and thought carefully about what I had written. Dr. Jo Eland, Associate Professor of Nursing at University of Iowa and a pioneer in the field of children's pain, gave good-humored support and contributed on her specialty TENS and acupressure. Dr. Christy Scott, with whom I thoroughly enjoyed teaching and working at BC Children's Hospital — and now miss since she has become an Assistant Professor at the School of Pharmacy, University of N. Carolina— co-wrote the sections on medication, acting as consultant on all matters pharmacological. Dr. Penny Leggott, now Associate Professor of Pediatric Dentistry in the School of Dentistry at the University of Washington, Seattle, demonstrated such gentle skill and fine timing with my own children in the chair that it was clear she was the dentist to co-write "Visiting the Dentist". Dr. Dan Kohen, Director, Behavioral Pediatrics Program at University of Minnesota in Minneapolis, my dear friend and colleague, with whom teaching workshops in Pediatric Hypnotherapy over many years still is a sheer delight, has a gift with the language of possibilities, and co-wrote the section on The Language that Helps Pain to Go in Chapter 6, and Emergency Pain.

I am deeply grateful to Dr Allan Basbaum of the Keck Science Institute of Integrative Studies at U. of Calif, San Francisco, for his generosity in sharing his writings with me. He was extraordinarily helpful with "How Pain Works" and helped make an initially intimating chapter a richly rewarding one to write. My warm thanks also to Dr. Joel Katz who thoughtfully commented on the completed chapter.

I am deeply appreciative for the help and involvement of the following:

- Family doctors for their comments on "Visiting the Doctor": Drs Sandy Witherspoon, Lalya Wickremasinghe, Charles King & Lori Smith; the patients at The Reach Clinic; Dr. Juergen Rauh for allowing us to photograph, and Nursing Professor Dr. Jackie Crisp, for her research on children's perspectives on invasive medical procedures.
- Pediatricians, Drs. Jane Hailey, Kevin Farrell, Tim Oberlander, Peter Malleson and Tony Richtsmeister who read, commented and guided me in areas requiring medical accuracy.
- My dear friends—colleagues from many disciplines, Physiotherapist, Occupational Therapist, Nurse, Biologist, Early Childhood Educator, Educator and Writer, Psychologist and Artist — most of whom are also parents, generously discussed, read and helped with different stages of the manuscript: Holly Andrews M.Ed., Dr. Susan Branson, Linda Bonnell R.N., Dr. Edna Durbach, Nuerit Fox M.Sc, Darby Honeyman BSc PT., Dr. Lesley Joy, Dr. David Pimm, Joanne Smith BSc OT, Cindy Stutzer MSN, Beryl Young, and Barbara Wood.
- Once the book was completed I turned to my trusted colleagues, Drs. Ken Craig, Gerri Frager, Naida Hyde, Helga Jacobson and Barbara Shapiro for their comments. I thank them for taking the time to go through the final manuscript, and for their constructive and thoughtful comments.
- My thanks also to Astra pharma Anne Taciuk, Linnea Steele, Martin Dash, Nancy Hale and Al Cook of Astra Pharma Inc. for giving me a grant to support a research assistant and photographer; to Mary Walsh (Ph.D. Cand.) my insightful and delightful research assistant;

to Lori Nemetz for her reseach; and to my talented photographer Kent Kallberg.

My skilled and highly intelligent editor Nancy Flight who came just at the right time, and quickly became invaluable to me. Her clear mind and sensitive editorial guidance ensured we had a readable book. My thanks also to Vic Marks and his staff for their assistance.

The children and parents with whom I've worked over the last 22 years have taught me the most. Many children and teenagers, particularly Jeremy Jacobson, Seanna Peterson, Shannon, Zack, Jodi, Tyler, and Michelle, contributed to this book by working with me, telling me their experiences and wanting their pain and anxiety to be better understood and managed so that their lives could be fun again. To all of those children and their families past, present, and future—my deep and abiding gratitude.